The Clinical Interview of the Child

Second Edition

About the Authors

Stanley I. Greenspan, M.D., is Clinical Professor of Psychiatry, Behavioral Sciences, and Pediatrics at the George Washington University Medical School, in Washington, D.C. Dr. Greenspan is also supervising Child Psychoanalyst at the Washington Psychoanalytic Institute. He was previously Chief of the Mental Health Study Center and Director of the Clinical Infant Development Program at the National Institute of Mental Health. A founder of the National Center for Clinical Infant Programs, Dr. Greenspan has been honored with a number of national awards, including the American Psychiatric Association's Ittleson Prize for outstanding contributions to child psychiatric research and the Strecker Award for outstanding contributions to American psychiatry. He is the author or editor of more than 15 books and 80 articles.

In addition to working on environmental issues, Nancy Thorndike Greenspan, a former health economist, writes about children's development.

The Clinical Interview of the Child

Second Edition

Stanley I. Greenspan, M.D.

with the collaboration of
Nancy Thorndike Greenspan

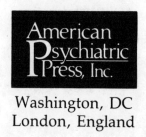

American Psychiatric Press, Inc.

Washington, DC
London, England

Note: The authors have worked to ensure that all information in this book concerning drug dosages, schedules, and routes of administration is accurate as of the time of publication and consistent with standards set by the U.S. Food and Drug Administration and the general medical community. As medical research and practice advance, however, therapeutic standards may change. For this reason and because human and mechanical errors sometimes occur, we recommend that readers follow the advice of a physician who is directly involved in their care or the care of a member of their family.

Books published by the American Psychiatric Press, Inc., represent the views and opinions of the individual authors and do not necessarily represent the policies and opinions of the Press or the American Psychiatric Association.

First Edition published by McGraw-Hill Book Company, 1981
Second Edition published by American Psychiatric Press, Inc., Copyright © 1991.

American Psychiatric Press, Inc.
1400 K Street, N.W., Washington, DC 20005

Library of Congress Cataloging-in-Publication Data

Greenspan, Stanley I.
    The clinical interview of the child / Stanley I. Greenspan, with the collaboration of Nancy Thorndike Greenspan.—2nd ed.
        p. cm.
    Includes bibliographical references and index.
    ISBN 0-88048-420-9
    1. Mental illness—Diagnosis.   2. Interviewing in child—
psychiatry.   3. Child psychology.   I. Greenspan, Stanley I.   II. Title.
    [DNLM: 1. Interview, Psychological—in infancy & childhood.
WS 105 G815c]
RJ503.G74   1991
618.92'89075—dc20
DNLM/DLC
for Library of Congress   90-14571
                                                                                    CIP

British Library Cataloguing in Publication Data

A CIP record is available from the British Library.

To our parents,
who began our education,
and our children, Elizabeth, Jake, and Sarah,
who enthusiastically continue it.

Contents

1

Conceptual Foundations: An Overview

THE CLINICAL INTERVIEW with the child presents an unusual challenge and opportunity. The challenge lies in the fact that children are complicated and yet, once their modes of communication are understood, at the same time straightforward. To the extent that the clinician is able to meet the challenge successfully, the clinical interview allows unique access to the child's highly individual world and special experiences, opening the way to accurate diagnosis and effective therapy.

Surprisingly enough, one of the main talents the clinician must possess is knowing how to stay out of the child's way as he reveals, at his own pace and in his own "words," the character and contents of his experiential world. At the same time the talented clinician will know when and how to step in and help the child communicate in an increasingly rich and personal manner. Being naturally ingenious, children will share their inclinations, thoughts, and feelings with the clinician through a variety of communication channels. The clinician's task is to be tuned in to all of these channels simultaneously and to be alert to every nuance of meaning conveyed.

The clinician must therefore be a highly skilled observer, a trait that includes seeing, hearing, and in other ways sensing all of the data the child provides. A basic requisite of being a good observer is to resist the very human tendency to jump to conclusions on the basis of insufficient evidence and thus propose premature formulations. Do not rush to explain your observations. Ask yourself questions and use hypotheses to test your understanding. Only when all the pertinent information is in should you formulate a diagnosis. Otherwise you may overlook important aspects of the child's personality.

As indicated, the basic requirement of a good clinician is the ability to observe in several dimensions simultaneously. Children communicate through the way they look at—or avoid looking at—the clinician, the style and depth of their personal relatedness, their gestures, their mood, the variety and types of emotions they manifest, the way they negotiate the space of the interview setting, the themes they develop in talk and play, and in many other ways as well. The organization, depth, age-appropriate relevance, and sequence of the child's affects and themes are all vehicles for sharing the structure, character, and contents of his or her experience. A good observer must therefore continuously monitor every communication channel—both verbal and nonverbal—that the child employs throughout their time together.

In the following chapters I will discuss in detail the principles and methods of systematic observation. I will then consider the way in which these observations lead to clinical judgments. Before turning to these practical matters, however, it will be useful to review a few general concepts of human behavior.

MULTIPLE LINES OF DEVELOPMENT

It is universally acknowledged among mental health professionals that personality develops along multiple lines. Development in the overall physical, neurological, cognitive, and intellectual realms, as well as the development of human relationships, coping strategies, and general styles of organizing and differentiating thoughts, wishes, and feelings—all these areas of development and more contribute to the ways one organizes and creates one's unique experience of life. Agreement on the most salient half-dozen areas could easily be reached; after that, various special frames of reference—e.g., social adaptation, family patterns—would augment the list differentially for various clinicians. The only disputes that arise in this general consensus about the multiplicity of developmental lines concern which proffered conceptualization helps us better understand human functioning. Some clinicians might emphasize the person's relationship to the external environment, the family, and other social structures; others might emphasize the person's intrapsychic, experiential world. Some might champion the primacy of the cognitive intellectual processes whereas others would favor the emotional processes. None would disagree, however, that each of these areas participates in the whole and demands consideration, particularly when one is trying to assess the total personality.

Unfortunately, theoretical acceptance of multiple lines of development is not matched by practical adherence, as is notable in many of our attempts at conducting the clinical examination—especially for research but also for clinical purposes. Thus too often an emphasis on the behavioral level is permitted to overshadow the experiential level, or a focus on the superficial aspects of social adaptation is allowed to exclude adequate consideration of how a person deals with deeply experienced feelings. An example will illustrate this point. Some young people who are class leaders, assertive and viewed by their peers and teachers as very competent, and who in general manifest behaviors consistent with highly successful and skillful social adaptation, may nevertheless develop severe depressions and even psychotic disorganizations. Some of these adolescents who were studied in depth were found to have had lifelong problems in handling certain deeply felt feelings involving passive longing, dependency, and intimacy. Insofar as the concept of multiple lines of development is paid lip service but not adhered to in a rigorous manner, clinical evaluations will tend to miss these subtler dimensions of human functioning.

To avoid being overwhelmed by complexities, clinical interviewers must have a conceptual framework that will alert them to the different dimensions of functioning that will emerge in the clinical setting. Anna Freud (1965) wrote an extraordinarily useful book, *Normality and Pathology in Childhood*, in which she delineated a number of developmental lines that can be useful in conceptualizing various dimensions of the child's behavior and experience. Likewise, Erik Erikson's (1950) work on the delineation of psychosocial stages, Margaret Mahler's (1975) work on the development and individuation of the self and the role of early object relations, and Jean Piaget's (1969) work on cognitive developmental stages are noteworthy contributions that delineate the developmental progression characteristic of different areas of personality functioning. More recently, clinical research studies of infants and young children have made it possible to formulate in greater detail the early stages in development and to observe how constitutional/maturational and experiential factors interact (Greenspan 1989).

The point I wish to underscore in introducing this volume is that a child's personality, no less than that of an adult, comprises many interrelated lines of development. It must also be remembered that, although these lines can be arbitrarily separated for conceptual purposes, in the functioning experience of a child they are all inter-related.

MULTIPLE DETERMINANTS OF BEHAVIOR

Another principle worthy of attention in these introductory comments is that every discrete behavior is multiply determined. In other words, when viewing human functioning it is an oversimplification or error to assume a one-to-one relationship between what is observed and some real or hypothesized causal factor.

For example, a child may be angry one day because a friend took his favorite game. He may be angry on another day because a girl flirted with him and he became sexually aroused. He may become angry at another time because he cannot understand the teacher's math instructions. On still another day he may be angry because his visiting grandparents have now gone home. And on yet another day he may be angry for all those reasons at once. This child may demonstrate his anger by throwing chalk at the blackboard on each of these occasions, and his chalk throwing may be the only behavior observed. Yet this single act of anger may be related to one of several different causes or to a combination of any number of them at a given time.

Similarly, a child may represent the same feeling or the same internal state with different behaviors. The child who feels angry in response to his father's belittling and making fun of him may behave provocatively. At another time, his reaction to this same type of humiliation may take the form of compliance and passivity. At still another time, he may behave competitively or in a disorganized way. Thus, an internal feeling of humiliation and anger may manifest itself in four or five different ways depending on the contextual situations or on other related internal states the child is experiencing.

In sum, this principle of multiple determination suggests that there are multiple relationships between what clinicians observe and the way children organize their experiential world.

THE DEVELOPMENTAL STRUCTURALIST APPROACH: A BRIEF SUMMARY

As one considers the multiple determinants of behavior and the multiple lines of development, it becomes increasingly necessary to have a model or a way of viewing development that is both sensitive to the complexities inherent in these concepts and useful to clinicians in their tasks of direct observation of children's experience. The developmental structuralist approach focuses on how a person organizes experience at each stage of development. Experience is broadly defined to encompass emotional experience as well as experience with the inanimate or impersonal world. The person's experiential organization is the final common pathway for multiple determinants (environmental, biological, etc.) that influence behavior and can be studied in relation to each specific line of development. The developmental structuralist approach, which is elaborated in *Intelligence and Adaptation* and *The Development of the Ego* (Greenspan 1979, 1989), will be only briefly discussed here.

Before describing this approach, it should be highlighted that for the reader not interested in theory, it is quite appropriate to skip this section and resume with Chapter 2. Two assumptions are related to this approach. One is that a person's organizational capacity progresses to higher levels as he or she matures. "Higher levels" in this context implies an ability to organize in stable patterns an increasingly wide and complex range of experience. The interplay between age-appropriate experience and maturation of the central nervous system ultimately determines the characteristics of this organizational capacity at each phase. The second assumption is that, for each phase of development, in addition to a characteristic organizational level, there are also certain characteristic types of experience (e.g., interests or inclinations) that "play themselves out," so to speak, within the organizational structure. Stage-specific experiences or inclinations are evidenced in the stage-specific types of wishes, fears, curiosities, and inclinations—often referred to as drives, psychosocial tasks, etc.[1] Stage-specific experiences are also related to the interplay of biological maturational processes and ongoing experience with the environment.

We therefore focus on *two* components of a person's experiential world. One component is the level of organization of experience. For example, we would expect an 8-year-old to organize her experience sufficiently to be able to separate reality from fantasy, modulate impulses, regulate mood, focus concentration, integrate thoughts and emotions, delineate—in an ever-subtler fashion—her sense of self from her sense of others, and maintain her self-esteem. The above abilities are the age-appropriate organizational features that characterize the adaptive experiential organization of an 8-year-old.

---

[1] The model being described here is a biological adaptational one, in that the adapting individual develops his or her unique experiential organizations and "contents" from an interplay in which maturational progression and its phase-specific inclinations operate on and are responded to by the environment.

In contrast, a maladaptive organization would be characterized by the tendency toward disorganization with vulnerable reality testing or impulse regulation.

The second component of a person's experiential world relates to the *type* of experience organized. Here one looks at the specific thoughts, concerns, inclinations, wishes, fears, and so forth. The type of experience is, in a sense, the drama the child is experiencing, whereas the organizational level might be viewed metaphorically as the stage on which this drama is being played. To carry this metaphor a step further, it is possible to imagine some stages that are large and stable and therefore can support a complex and intense drama. In comparison, other stages may be narrow or small and thus able to contain only a very restricted drama. Still other stages may have cracks in them or crumble easily under the pressure of an intense, rich, and varied drama.

According to the developmental structuralist approach, at each phase of development there are certain characteristics that define the experiential organizational capacity, i.e., the stability and contour of the stage. At the same time there are certain age-appropriate dramas or themes characterized by their complexity, richness, depth, and content. This approach then provides a set of expectations and clinical-indicator behaviors or capacities for each age or developmental stage. It focuses on adaptive capacities expected as well as on limitations and conflicts.

THE FOUR ORGANIZATIONAL LEVELS OF DEVELOPMENT

Consider four organizational levels of development. These four levels are derived from the six stages of ego development postulated and discussed in some detail elsewhere (Greenspan 1989). The six stages of ego development were formulated through observation and clinical work with normal and disturbed infants, young children, and their families. It was observed that experience was organized along adaptive or maladaptive dimensions in relationship to a series of specific developmental challenges. These six developmental challenges can be condensed into four core processes, or levels. They involve how a child 1) attends and engages, 2) communicates with gestures and behaviors, 3) creates internal mental images (ideas) and shares them with others (i.e., symbols, mental representations), and 4) categorizes these meanings and makes connections between them.

The first level, which comes from the two stages of regulation and interest in the world and attachment, involves *engagement*, which has two components—*shared attention* and *engagement*. Not infrequently clinicians try to get a "tuned-out," inattentive child to verbalize rather than first simply to attend. Attention depends in part on the ability to take in information through each sensory modality. Overreactivity, underreactivity, or processing difficulties in any sensory pathway will affect attention. Muscle tone, motor coordination, and motor planning will also influence attention.

Engagement, or a sense of relatedness, requires that both parties feel connected to each other. This sounds self-evident. But frequently the clinician ignores the quality of engagement so that indifference, negative feelings, or impersonal or aloof patterns continue longer than necessary.

The second organizational level is derived from the two stages of purposeful communication and an organized, complex sense of self. It involves organized patterns of behavior and *intentional, nonverbal communication (i.e., gestures)*. These gestures include facial expressions, sounds, posture, arm and leg movements, and so forth. From the middle of the first year of life onward, individuals are always using gestures to communicate. The basic emotional messages of life— safety and security versus danger, acceptance versus rejection, approval versus disapproval—are all communicated through facial expressions, body posture, movement patterns, and vocal tone and rhythm. Words enhance these more basic communications, but interestingly we all form quick, split-second judgments regarding new persons' dangerousness, safety or rejection, or acceptance of us from their gestures before the conversation even gets started. In fact, if a person looks dangerous and says, "You know I am quite safe," we tend to believe the gestures and disbelieve the words.

At a more subtle level, gestural communication also relays to us what aspects of our own emotions are being accepted, ignored, or rejected. The looks and head nods as we communicate about closeness, curiosity, anger, or excitement quickly tell us how the person feels about our message. More importantly, our emerging definition of the uniqueness of our very self is dependent on how others react to our own special tendencies with preverbal gestures. Differential responses are part of the process that refines and defines our emerging behavior and sense of self. How is our mischievous behavior and smile responded to—with a smile and grin of acceptance or a headshaking frown of disapproval? Our natural inclinations are in part either accepted and supported or refined as part of this nonverbal communication system. Over time, gestural communication helps the child organize more and more complex behavior and an emerging sense of self.

The clinician who focuses only on a child's words or intellectual abilities will often miss the lack of organized gestural communication. For example, the child who marches to his own drummer, floats in and out of the room, does not respond to the parent's facial expressions and sounds with his own facial expressions and sounds (each and every time), or does not follow the parent's arm and hand gestures with his own shows a lack of organized gestural communication.

Similarly, clinicians often focus on changing isolated behaviors or symptoms and ignore the foundation needed for interpersonal processes. The child may, in fact, be missing the very process of interchange that goes on every second that two people are near each other and that binds people together in an organized, intentional manner. Organized, interactive communication, rather than isolated skills, is the foundation for language reasoning and emotional adaptation. The ability to organize behavior and emotions and to communicate intentionally with gestures and behavior go hand in hand and help the child integrate and comprehend the world.

The third and fourth organizational levels come from the stages of representational *elaboration* and *differentiation*. The third level involves the elaboration and sharing of meanings. The functional and interactive use of words and pretend or symbolic play is used interactively to communicate wishes or intentions, feelings, and thoughts. At the fourth level, shared meanings are used both to elaborate wishes and feelings, as in pretend play, and to categorize meanings and solve problems, as in logical conversations. At this level, the child can make connections between different ideas or feelings ("I am mad because you took my toy") and balance fantasy and reality.

Shared meanings involve the communication of ideas, not just having ideas. Some children are great at pretend play and talking, but only communicate their own ideas, never building on the responses of the other person. They talk and they play out dramas, but they do not easily take in or use someone else's ideas and comments. For example, whenever Sally came home from preschool, she played out scene after scene of being a queen, letting mother hold her cape, but not answering or even reflecting on minor questions about the play like, "What does the queen want me to do next?" or about her day, "How did school go?" or "Who did you play with today?" Other children are just the opposite, diligently following the parents' instructions, listening to every word, but rarely elaborating their own understanding of events.

Children are only capable of the levels they have gone through. By 18 months, the child should have mastered the first two levels, and by age 3½, all four levels.

These four organizational levels are easy to observe, but often are taken for granted. The child comes into the playroom ready to play or talk. There is often some rapport or some emotional relatedness that develops—hence, the stage of engagement. As soon as the therapist opens the door and the child goes to the toys as the therapist's gestures suggest, or they make eye contact, with perhaps a few facial or arm gestures, we have an intentional, preverbal communication system going. (Of course, some children may already evidence some difficulty in the preverbal communication system, or even at the earlier level of engagement. But many establish these first two levels rather easily.) As the child begins complex play, such as crashing cars, or making sounds and pointing to indicate "get me that," we have more complex intentional communication. When the child puts feelings into words and elaborates pretend play themes, the third level is reached—the level of shared meanings (representational elaboration). The fourth level will be reached when the child not only elaborates themes, but constructs bridges between domains of experience—"I'm scared when I'm mad"). The ability to categorize experience also indicates representational differentiation: There is now a symbolic "me" and a symbolic "you" and "I always get so scared of everything." Most importantly, the capacity for categorizing experience helps the patient elaborate feelings and build on another's communications. The child can have a logical two-way dialogue and tell the difference between fantasy and reality.

Children may have clear compromises in their attainment of these organizational levels, such as the child who comes in and can only partially engage. When anxious or frightened this child quickly disengages and becomes aloof or withdrawn. Also, let us consider that at the same time this child gets disorganized and can't even gesture purposefully and intentionally (e.g., he gestures and talks in a disorganized way). His capacity for representational elaboration is limited to either disorganized emotional communications or organized descriptions of impersonal events. There is little capacity for balancing subjective elaborations and an appreciation of reality. This child then uses words in a fragmented way, tends to be concrete and impersonal in his descriptions of the world, gesturally signals in a disorganized and chaotic way and, while capable of engaging with others, easily disengages and becomes aloof.

To visualize this approach, picture these four levels: engagement; purposeful, organized communication; shared meanings; and categorized meanings. Then visualize alongside each level the different affective-thematic domains that characterize the human drama. These may include dependency, pleasure, assertiveness, curiosity, anger, self-limit-setting, empathy, and more consistent forms of love.

One can then look at which themes can be communicated at a given level. For example, a child may be able to use gestures but not representations to communicate dependency or love, i.e., he can't say, "I love you" or "hug me" and can't use dolls to play out a scene of two dolls hugging. He is, however, quite capable of physically hugging his mother and making loving facial expressions and sounds.

It should be pointed out that the fourth level becomes further developed in terms of extended representational systems and additional tasks or challenges, such as triangular relationships, the peer group, and forming values and ideals. These are discussed in detail elsewhere (Greenspan 1979).

Specific Lines of Development

Each organizational level and type of experience may be studied in relation to a number of different lines of development. Abstract notions can thereby be brought down to a concrete level, particularly if the lines of development one chooses have directly observable clinical referents. For example, in looking at physical and neurological development, one may study the child's development of gross motor capacities, fine motor capacities, perceptual-motor coordinating capacities, higher-level central nervous system integrative capacities, and particular stylistic preferences at different ages. One can see, for example, how the motor system can be used for or can undermine engagement or intentionality. The landmarks for adaptive and maladaptive patterns are well known (and will be described later in Chapter 3).

In looking at organizational levels, one may also consider the development of human relationships. The infant progresses from a general interest in both the inanimate and the human world, to a specific and preferred interest in primary caretakers (engagement), to a capacity to be intentional with and differentiate the primary caretakers from others, to an ability to relate to the primary caretakers with a deepening sense of pleasure as well as protest and assertion. We observe, for example, the toddler develop—as part of his or her unfolding relationship capacities—the ability to communicate through complex gestures desires for closeness, intimacy, and dependency and an interest in curious, independent, assertive exploration of the world. It is also possible to delineate the age-appropriate organizational levels and unique experiential patterns for such affects as anxiety, and thematic communication capacities.

It is important to keep in mind the distinction between the child's capacity for a certain organizational level along each developmental line and the child's particular experiential orientation—the content of his or her particular drama. For example, one possibility is for the child to achieve a level of development in human relationships where dependency and intimacy can be organized in a balanced and harmonious way with tendencies toward independence, mastery, and exploration: witness the 15-month-old toddler who can joyfully explore the rooms in the house alone and then comfortably return to mother or father or other primary caretakers for pleasurable, secure interchanges (or at times not so pleasurable, but nonetheless intimate interchanges).

In contrast, another child may be totally chaotic and fragmented, with no purposefulness, or can only experience clinging dependency, holding onto mother's or father's leg and refusing to explore the world; still another child may be impervious to mother, father, and other people and seems only to explore the inanimate world with a calm, almost bland, resolve that leads the observer to question the level of interest or pleasure this child is experiencing.

A determination should be made about the range of experience a child can organize before the drama that child may choose to play out is considered. The first child, who is capable of integrating within his experiential organization (in terms of the line of development concerned with human relationships) intimacy as well as some relative independence, may choose or show a preference for a drama that has to do with zooming cars. Another child may show preference for a drama that has to do with dolls falling off chairs or with peekaboo games. While the particular drama—the contents of the child's communications or play—is very interesting and important, it should not be confused with an independent determination of the child's organizational level of experience. While there *are* characteristic dramas or themes that tend to reflect certain phases of development, it is important to point out that the content of the dramas varies widely because it is determined by both experiential (environmental) and biological factors. Nonetheless, if one constructs categories broadly enough, one does tend to see general trends characteristic of different levels of organization. The relative universality of the Oedipal drama would be an example of such a trend.

Abstracted Formulations

As suggested above, the organizational level as well as the particular types of experience a child embraces can be delineated for each separate developmental line. At a descriptive level, looking at the child's physical and neurological capacities and inclinations, relationships, affects and emotions, thematic communication patterns, and so forth affords a very well-discriminated, detailed view of the child.

At the same time the developmental structuralist model also lends itself to abstracting from these highly detailed observations of the child's organizational level and experiential orientation in each line, categories reflecting overall developmental status. These categories of functioning may be viewed on a spectrum from maladaptive to adaptive organizational patterns. At one extreme, for example, there are defects in organizational integrity. A determination of a personality defect would be made when there is a severe impairment in the age-appropriate level of "core" personality or ego functions, such as reality testing, mood regulation, or impulse modulation. Such defects in the ability to organize experience according to age-appropriate levels often occur in relation to faulty development in the first 3 to 4 years of life when such basic organizational capacities are being developed. The specific types of defects that stem from faulty development at each period of early development will be discussed in detail later.

Another level of maladaptive development may be summarized under the category of constrictions in the flexibility of the personality. In this category there are no major defects in age-appropriate organizational capacities, but the range of experience that can be organized is restricted. For example, a 5-year-old child may have the capacity to test reality, but only in the context of very impersonal, shallow relationships and with affects of low intensity or affects restricted to the aggressive or negativistic domains. To use the metaphor of the stage and drama again, the stage does not have cracks in it and is not vulnerable to crumbling, but is extraordinarily narrow and therefore accommodates only a very restricted drama.

We may see restrictions ranging from severe ones based on compromises made early in life to minor ones stemming from later compromises. For example, there is a difference between persons who can maintain the integrity of their organizational capacities (the capacity for reality testing) only by totally walling off all human intimacy, and those who have minor limitations in experiencing assertive feelings with authority figures but otherwise function in an adaptive, age-appropriate way. The latter type of child simply may not be able to compete fully, whereas the former type of child realizes only a shadow of his or her human potential. The various types of constrictions will be described later (e.g., limiting the experience of certain types of feelings or thoughts, externalizing internal experiences).

A third, very subtle type of constrictive impairment is called an *encapsulated disorder*, based on the child's inability to maintain experiential continuity over time in narrowly delineated areas of experience, only minimally compromising the overall age-appropriate flexibility of personality (e.g., avoiding assertiveness only with authority figures that are very similar to one's father).

Once a judgment is made about the child's level and type of organizational defect and/or constriction, one can then categorize the type of drama being played out. Dramas, some of which are quite painful, may play themselves out in age-appropriate experiential organizations (e.g., phase-specific conflicts); less painful dramas may play themselves out in very constricted or even defective organizations.

In summary, experience may be organized at different levels; each level may have its own stylistic uniqueness; and each line of human development (delineated according to clinically meaningful categories) may be described in terms of its organizational level and its experiential uniqueness. Detailed observations of each line of development may be abstracted into a formulation about the overall level of personality functioning in terms of personality defects and constrictions, as well as adaptive, age-appropriate patterns.

The Developmental Structuralist Approach in Other Models of Development

The developmental structuralist approach, which focuses attention on the organization and content of experience, is compatible with most models of human behavior. For example, in psychoanalytic or psychodynamic approaches, the focus on dynamic, structural, genetic, and ego-psychological perspectives is related to the maturational and experiential properties of the personality. For example, the dynamic perspective focuses on the relationship of a person's drives or wishes to the fears, internalized prohibitions, reality constraints, and defense mechanisms of the personality. The dynamic perspective therefore becomes a "window" through which to study certain unique experiences. The genetic perspective orients us toward the historical unfolding of dynamic trends and is consistent with the biological adaptational approach suggested earlier. The structural and ego-psychological perspectives, which also focus our attention on conflict, alert us to the mediating properties of the ego—its ability to synthesize the person's drives or wishes, fears, internalized prohibitions, and reality considerations. The ego's defensive operations and integrating and synthesizing capacities can be studied from this perspective.

Psychodynamic approaches also embrace object-relations theory. Object-relations theory formulates the way early relationship patterns are internalized into self- and object representations, and how these internalizations form the foundation for basic personality functions. Object-relations theory explains how certain organizational capacities of the personality are achieved.

This very brief overview is provided to suggest that the theoretical perspective of this work is compatible with and encompasses important psychodynamic viewpoints, and thus orients the skilled clinician to a microscopic examination of the organizational level and experiential uniqueness of the child.

At another extreme are behavioral and behavioral-learning approaches. These approaches, which focus on observable behavior rather than on internal experience, and on the environmental factors that appear to influence behavior through their contextual or temporal relationship to behavior, seem to be diametrically opposed to psychodynamic perspectives . Quite to the contrary, they provide a complementary orientation whose theoretical rationale I have described elsewhere (Greenspan 1975).

In considering behavioral approaches, which are highly focused on environmental influences, it should be emphasized that a developmental model is needed to understand both the behavioral repertoire of the growing child at each phase of development and the likelihood that certain events will be experienced as reinforcing. Children are not simply a product of what they experience at any moment in time—or of past experiences, for that matter—but rather, of their capacities to *organize* experience at certain levels. The model presented here, which attempts to delineate the particular way children organize experience at each level of development, in a sense provides a picture of age-appropriate behavioral repertoires and potential categories of reinforcing events—or to put it more broadly, experiential repertoires.

In behavioral learning terms, these experiential repertoires can be viewed from the perspective of their organizational level and "content" uniqueness. For example, in using a behavioral learning approach with a child one first needs to make a determination regarding which categories of behavior to change. One does not wish to help a passive child be more assertive when that child has a more fundamental difficulty in behaving realistically. In other words, if a child has a defect in the organizational capacity for reality testing— which at a behavioral level emerges through a tendency to behave unrealistically—that issue may require attention first. If the clinician misses the child's fundamental difficulty in "behaving realistically" because he or she lacks a conceptual framework for finding clinically relevant categories of behavior, the treatment approach that is formulated may exacerbate, rather than alleviate, the child's primary difficulty. For example, a child may become more fragmented and unrealistic as she behaves more assertively. The developmental structuralist approach therefore is not only compatible with behavioral approaches, but may aid in delineating the most clinically relevant "experiential" categories.

Empirical Aspects of a Developmental Structuralist Approach

The developmental structuralist approach, though tied to a cohesive theory (see Greenspan 1979, 1989), can also be used in an atheoretical, empirical manner. In a sense, the identification of the ways children organize experience and their phase-specific stylistic uniqueness at each level of development may be documented without regard to a particular theory. The observational categories described in Chapter 2 can be judged on their own merits in terms of their usefulness for clinical evaluation, planning, and following the course of treatment. The "acid test" would be their usefulness in a variety of research contexts: describing stage-specific behavior and making predictions about future behavior, predicting the treatment approaches likely to be effective with certain types of problems and individuals, etc. In other words, the validity of this approach can be empirically assessed by its application in a variety of clinical and research contexts.

Relationship of the Developmental Structuralist Approach to Traditional Diagnostic Categories

As will be suggested later, the developmental structuralist approach can be used in conjunction with existing standard diagnostic categories. The existing diagnostic scheme of the American Psychiatric Association DSM-III-R (American Psychiatric Association 1987) does not attempt a cohesive developmental focus that encompasses multiple developmental lines. It takes into account certain syndromes of childhood. It tends to base these syndromes either on symptom clusters, personality traits, or an identification of etiological factors. For example, Axes I and II in the DSM-III-R approach, which focus on the syndromes and personality types, are not tied to a cohesive theory of human development that considers adaptation and maladaptation at each developmental level along a number of clinically relevant lines.

The developmental approach suggested here offers a potentially useful addition—a way to understand each child in terms of his or her developmental tendencies for each area of functioning.

One may use the approach suggested here as a complement to the traditional diagnostic categories. As will be described later, one may consider a three-column approach, where symptom clustering and personality-trait-oriented diagnostic labels (Axes I and II from

DSM-III-R) are represented in one column. In another column, diagnoses based on etiological factors may be represented (such diagnoses are rare, but are important to list when they are known—these are usually contained in Axis I). In yet a third column, one may list a developmental diagnosis based on how children organize and delineate their experiential world. We will see that developmental diagnoses are meaningful not only for diagnostic purposes but for clinical evaluation and planning, as well as for understanding etiological factors. Interventions that are based on symptoms, etiological factors, and developmental understanding of how a child negotiates and organizes his or her experiential world will be more complete in the way they help a child move ahead in his or her development than when based on only one or another set of factors in isolation.

GENERAL PRINCIPLES

I began with the principles of multiple determinants of behavior and multiple lines of development—and suggested that we use the developmental structuralist model to explore these principles—in order to emphasize just how complex our task is in the clinical interview of a child. We are asked to determine not only what is troubling a child at a particular point in his or her development but also to understand the child's personality organization. The problem for an 8-year-old boy, for example, might be that he has conflicts with his mother, who is trying to keep him dependent while he wishes to move out and do more things on his own. Perhaps the boy is being negativistic and belligerent, and not working in school, and so comes in for an assessment.

Here, you not only have to assess the nature of the problem that precipitated the visit, but you are also asked to assess any other issues that may be related. Even more important, you are also called on to assess the structure in which this current difficulty is occurring. How is this child functioning across the board, what kind of psychological or personality organization has this child achieved, and how does this organization compare with age-appropriate expectations? In other words, you are called on to make an assessment along multiple developmental lines, to describe the theater or stage, as it were, in which the current drama is being played out. To use a medical analogy, a physician needs to know the basic state of the patient's health before treating an infection. Treating an infection in a person with another chronic condition such as cancer is very different from treating an infection in a person who is otherwise healthy.

Mastering the complexity of the clinical diagnostic situation requires rigorous observation and conceptualization combined with patience. We must avoid the temptation to become too simplified in our approaches as a defense against our sense of just how complex life is in our area of work. One may throw up one's hands and say, If life is so complicated, if human beings are so complex in their functioning, and if the interview of the child demands that I be aware of multiple lines of development and multiple determinants of behavior, how am I ever to conclude anything? But rather than causing one to give up in despair, the complexity of human functioning should inspire the novice as well as the skilled clinician to rise to the occasion. The challenge will not be met with premature formulations or a narrowed focus that encompasses only a few dimensions of experience. Moreover, in the context of the clinical interview, the current vogue for too much operationalizing and quantifying of human behavior must be viewed as inconsistent with the processes necessary for a full understanding of the child's functioning.

The challenge presented by the clinical interview of the child can be met with an approach that is geared to unraveling complexity. In brief, interviewers must train themselves to monitor the multiple channels of communication used by the child; the data obtained will generate hypotheses that, through a process of gradual approximation, will clarify the problem at hand. In the succeeding chapters I outline the framework for simultaneously observing multiple dimensions of human functioning during the clinical interview, and describe, first, how to translate these observations into first-order clinical inferences and then how to derive clinical hypotheses and judgments from these inferences.

2

Framework for Systematic Observation of the Child

In THIS CHAPTER, I detail a number of categories for observation during the interview. These categories elaborate the concept of general organizational levels, described in Chapter 1, in relation to different dimensions of development such as relationships, affects, and themes. Specific contexts, such as relationship styles or specific affects or unique thematic fantasies, can then be considered for each category at each age or developmental level. These categories are presented through age 10.

In each category, two levels of data are pertinent. One is the descriptive level; that is, accurate description of the observed behavior. The other is the age-appropriate level; that is, an assessor must have some sense of the age- or developmental stage–appropriate functioning for each of these categories so that departures from the range can be noticed.

The first category includes everything related to the physical integrity of the child. The next category involves the emotional tone of the child during the assessment. The third category concerns how the child relates to you as a human being during the interview. The fourth concerns the specific affects and anxieties that become elaborated during the initial clinical interview. The fifth category covers the way the child uses the environment of the waiting room and the playroom. The sixth deals with thematic development: the way the child develops themes in terms of depth, richness, organization, and— of great importance—sequence. The final category covers your subjective feelings—the reaction of the diagnostician to the child. The data in this last category concern the feelings the child evokes in you— both your general feelings at the end of the interview and any specific fantasies or feelings you experienced during the interview. These first-order observations should yield good data, and good data are basic to any hypotheses you may formulate.

Let me add that, although the examples that follow refer to an interview playroom setting, these observational categories can be used in any setting. A child on an inpatient unit or in a schoolroom, for example, can be observed from these multiple perspectives. You can notice how he relates to the other children, how he uses you, how he uses space, his physical and neurological status in terms of activity level and coordination, and his mood and changing affects during the observation period. Although systematic observation is easier when you have a child alone—such as in a playroom session or in your own interview setting—it can be done in any setting. A teacher in a schoolroom can use this observational framework as effectively as a nurse on a hospital ward.

PHYSICAL AND NEUROLOGICAL DEVELOPMENT

Let us now discuss each of the above-mentioned categories in detail, beginning with physical and neurological development. Here, you want to observe the level of the child's physical and neurological intactness in order to determine if further neurological or psychological assessment is needed. You can begin observation in the waiting room when you greet the child. You notice things like the child's posture, gait, balance, fine motor coordination, gross motor coordination, speech, and quality and tone of voice. You want to get any impression you can about the child's sensory system (DeGangi and Greenspan 1988a, 1988b, 1989; Greenspan 1989). Does the child have any difficulty in hearing you or seeing you, any difficulty in experiencing sensations through touch?

You also want to observe if the child is over- or underreactive to any sensations (e.g., sound or touch) or has difficulty processing sensation in one or another modality (e.g., can't sequence your words). Children can be over- or underreactive to any sensations—sounds, sights, touch, their own movements. Careful observation will reveal if a physical, maturational, individual difference or an emotional factor, or aspects of both, are involved in, for example, a child's being cautious about physical closeness. In addition, careful observations will reveal auditory-verbal or visual-spatial processing difficulties. For example, the child who doesn't respond to your gestures or words with gestures or words of her own should not be assumed to be emotionally preoccupied or globally distractible. There may be a specific processing difficulty.

You also want to look for sensorimotor and gross and fine motor coordination. Is this a clumsy child who has trouble integrating body movements? When you shake the child's hand, you can see how he meets your hand and whether he has good hand-eye coordination. By watching the gait, you can see if certain large muscle groups and gross motor functioning are intact. Once in the playroom or interview setting, there will be an opportunity to see fine motor coordination when the child draws or colors. If the child avoids that material, at some point in the interview you might suggest drawing in order to see his fine motor coordination.

You want to look at the child's overall physical well-being in terms of height, weight, skin tone, and general health. You should observe the activity level of the child, not only at the beginning of the interview but throughout it. Is this a child who shows some variation in activity level around certain tasks—does she get excited or involved and then slow down and concentrate? Is the child extremely active and uncontrollable from the beginning of the interview, or very slow and passive in all activity? How does the child attend? Can she focus on you, on toys, on games or drawings? How does her attention in the office compare to reports or observations of her behavior in groups, such as at school? All these things you can observe at the beginning of the hour to get an initial impression, and then continue observing throughout the hour, noting any changes. Such changes are important, particularly if you want to make an assessment of a functional cause of some physical difficulty. With a child who has a questionable learning difficulty, for example, you may find that, though initially fine motor coordination and sensorimotor integration look good, when you hit on some anxiety-arousing area, all of a sudden the child falls apart. Such data suggest that some issues in the emotional sphere interfere with certain physical capabilities.

One can perform a very general neurological examination without laying hands on the child. There is much to be observed about the functioning of the physical and neurological systems. For instance, if you observe some spasticity you can wonder about cerebral palsy of a minor nature without having to test the child's reflexes. If you notice any unusual weaknesses in a limb or on one side of the body, you should again be thinking in this way. Some psychiatrists may wish to conduct their own general neurological examination, whereas others will form impressions based on their observations and make an appropriate referral when indicated. Questioning the family about the child's development will help determine whether a neurological evaluation is necessary.

In another case, you may decide that psychological evaluation is necessary. For example, after you have entered the waiting room and introduced yourself to an 8-year-old girl, she jumps and skips back into the playroom, where she socks a bag a couple of times. When it comes to drawing, however, her fine motor coordination seems to be immature. Although she is 8 years old, she has trouble making letters. These observations may raise questions about whether there is some central nervous system immaturity or minimal dysfunction; you may want psychological testing to focus on this area.

In summary, even in your initial session you can reach the determination of whether a neurological workup is necessary, and what specific work you wish to have done in areas where you have questions. You should have a fairly good idea whether the psychological test results (e.g., the developmental level on the Bender Visual Motor Gestalt Test) are going to tell you something, and if you are surprised by them it should raise a diagnostic question. In other words, if you see a child whose physical and neurological integrity seem intact but whose developmental level on the Bender is very immature, you want to know why there is a discrepancy between your clinical observations and the test results.

MOOD

The next category deals with the mood or overall emotional tone. From the very beginning, you want to notice the child's mood, and then you want to watch how it evolves during the interview. It is different from the variations in affect or emotion that you will see throughout the interview. Your perception of the mood or general emotional tone will be an integrated judgment based on the way the child looks and behaves as well as on the content of his or her speech. Looking at mood from outside the clinical context for a moment, you may feel that a friend is depressed, based on observation of many aspects of that person's behavior. The person may talk about happy events but look sad, move sluggishly, and make occasional veiled comments about whether life is worth living. Taken all together, your observations indicate that the person is depressed.

In determining the child's mood, you should use any behavioral references you have to construct an overall picture. Facial expression is a good example. You can see if the child is sad-looking, sits in a corner, and is not involved with anyone in the waiting room; or if the child is cheerful, a little hypermanic, and optimistic about the world. Often the mood you perceive is an intuitive impression because children rarely show certain moods (depression is an example) that are obvious in teenagers or adults.

The content of the interview is also relevant to the assessment of the mood. If you meet a sad, lonely-looking, 5-year-old girl who shakes hands limply, walks in passively and sits inertly, and then finally begins playing out themes involving destruction, you know that content supports the observations you have gathered about emotional tone or mood. If the child's themes evolve to feelings of helplessness—no matter how hard she tries, nothing goes right for her—the evidence is consistent with the overall mood.

Your own subjective feeling at the end of an interview can be extremely helpful in assessing a child's mood. Some leave you feeling depressed, and it is important not to rationalize and disregard your feeling by thinking, for example, Well, I'm tired, it's been a long day, or, I had a fight with my spouse earlier in the day. Other children leave you feeling invigorated, which is also a diagnostic clue. The seductive child who invigorates you; the sad, hungry child who leaves you feeling drained; and other children who evoke various other feelings—each child provides clues about mood by means of your subjective response. Any discrepancy between your observations and your subjective response may indicate that the overall emotional tone of the child is more complicated than it appears. You may want to have a second or a third diagnostic session, depending on how many questions remain unanswered after your first session.

HUMAN RELATIONSHIP CAPACITY

The next category, relatedness to other persons, involves an examination of how the child relates to you. While you are with the child, you should observe how he or she treats you as a person, how your relationship develops, and how differentiated it is. As is true for all these categories, observations belonging to this category begin in the waiting room. As you enter the waiting room and relax for a minute between patients, you want to observe both the interaction between the child and whoever brought him and between the child and others in the room. Is he being affectionate, or withdrawn and aloof? Is he making contact with others; how much distance does he maintain from them? Simply by watching for half a minute or so, you get an impression of how the child has negotiated all the available human relationships in the waiting room.

Do not dismiss from consideration or excuse on situational grounds what the child has chosen to do. If you see a child who is clinging for dear life to mother's hand, ignoring the other adults and the playthings in the waiting area, you might wonder to yourself if this child is scared to death of coming to the hospital or office and seeing a psychiatrist. This snap impression should always take the form of a hypothesis. It is a mistake to formulate explanations so early in the clinical meeting. Do not fall into the trap of trying to explain the behavior before you have all the data.

While you are in the waiting room, it is also important to note your initial reaction to the family. With one family, we feel comfortable nodding to the mother and standing and observing for a few minutes, just relaxing between patients; we see no display of discomfort in the family. With another family, however, we find that as soon as they see us, we feel compelled to go to them immediately; we cannot relax for a minute or take a few deep breaths between patients. We experience such a family as demanding our immediate attention and we are anxious to comply, as if we sense that they will be insulted and angry if we do not. Use this intuition as another clue to what is going on—even if you react to it, which is sometimes appropriate so as not to put too much stress on a family during a diagnostic phase.

After observing how the child relates to the people in the waiting room and what your reaction to the family is, you should note how the child relates to you, human being to human being. How does the child greet you? Is she wide-eyed, asking how you are, eager to come along with you? Or, as soon as you enter, does the child run to the other side of the room, greet you with some caution and apprehension, yet show a willingness to come along, enough trust to come into the playroom without mother? Or does the child start crying and fussing, hold on to mother's leg, and demand that she come into the playroom with her? What is the first feeling tone between the two of you as people? Is it a twinkle of acceptance in the child's eye, but with some anxious glances toward mother, thus showing you a combination of interest and apprehension?

It is the extremes that should be noticed here. You cannot expect to appreciate subtleties in a few minutes, but you can certainly pick up on the aloof, distant child who does not want to make contact with you at all. Such observations will give you clues about the areas you may want to explore. For example, I remember seeing one 3-

year-old girl who took my hand as if I were a long-lost favorite uncle she had been waiting to see. I felt good, because so many children greet one quite differently. But the way this child took my hand and came skipping along to the playroom made me feel almost too tremendously accepted. She did not show the normal wariness of a stranger. Subsequently this behavior proved to be a clue to the fact that the child was emotionally promiscuous in relating to people. You will see this kind of global emotional hunger and lack of discrimination in relating to people in some children with a history of early deprivation.

As you gain experience, you will get a sense of the initial types of behavior acceptable from a new patient—child or adult. Often the first tip-off to a borderline or psychotic problem occurs in the first few minutes of the interview when the child does something that you cannot quite identify because it is outside the realm of normal, acceptable opening moves. (Of course, "acceptable" opening moves are not delineated as such, but your intuition tells you something is amiss.) Again, having an unusual feeling is a clue to a diagnostic *question*, rather than an indication of any conclusion.

Once the interview begins, does the child make contact with you at a personal level? Do you feel a personal sense of relatedness? Does that sense evolve, and at what point? Does the relatedness vary throughout the interview? Take a normal, healthy 6½-year-old child who may have some circumscribed neurotic problem. We might expect the child to start out cautiously, maybe warily, because you are a new person in his or her life. You may expect the child to warm up to you slowly during the interview; you will feel a sense of relatedness evolving. You will get a sense of this child as another human being. You will not feel that there is a mechanical quality or a distant, "not all there" quality. You will not feel an impersonal kind of hunger wherein the child regards and uses you as if you were just another object in the room like the guns or the toy animals. Instead, you feel a relationship beginning as you find yourself getting more interested in this child. By the end of the hour, different emotions and themes emerge and the relationship grows. You will feel that the two of you have made some emotional contact.

This prototypical child might be compared with one who is persistently aloof and emotionally detached, never making contact with you. Such a child may keep his back to you and maintain a distance of 6 or 7 feet from you. He may be interested in some of the inanimate objects and games, he may even talk or look at you, but you never feel any sense of relatedness. A third type is the child who wants you to be there all the time, who is hungry for any human attention and involves you in everything.

In addition, you may observe subtler ways in which the child

relates to you as a person, ways that are suggestive of certain characterological traits. For instance, you may see the child who wants
to control you. As the interview begins, you get a sense of human
relatedness, but then the child tries to control you. He or she gives
you orders, has you play this game or that. You make a suggestion
because you want to see the youngster draw. The child replies, "No,
we are going to do this now," showing an orderly kind of obsessive
behavior. Other boys and girls may be seductive and flirtatious in the
way they engage you. You find yourself not only getting interested
but even a little excited. You find you are enjoying yourself thor-
oughly, and if you allow them to continue, you may have some
interesting fantasies. This kind of seductiveness is usually thought to
happen across sexes in Oedipal-aged children: the boy will be seductive with the female interviewer, the girl with the male interviewer. But the same thing can also happen when therapist and child
are of the same sex. Whatever the case, such observations will give
you a clue to the child's style of relating.

Experience with many children will give you the basis to look
with sensitivity at the nature of the relationship. A set of internal,
intuitive norms will evolve for you.

Let us take the example of a child who starts by showing
slight apprehension. First he glances tentatively at mother. Then he
comes into the room, sits in the corner for a minute or two, and asks
whether he can play with something. You nod approval, and he
begins exploring the room. Through play his fantasy about children
having operations in hospitals emerges. You make a comment, "I
understand that kids can be scared that when they come to a hospital,
they are going to get operated on." The boy looks frightened for a
second and begins taking the dolls and playing out a drama with one
doll operating on another doll.

Shortly thereafter, you suddenly sense the child moving closer
to you, shortening by half the 8-foot distance he had been keeping.
He begins inviting you to get involved in play with him, whereas
before he played alone. He wants you to manipulate one of the dolls
for him. You begin feeling more comfortable and the sense of apprehension diminishes. In this example, then, you have seen some growth
and development in relatedness during the interview: from tentativeness, fear, and wariness, to an elaboration of concerns that most
people have with any new person, and then to some beginning sense
of warmth. This particular scenario may be suggestive of a fairly well-
integrated child.

An example of an opposite sequence may go something like
this: The child starts off being intimate and close, comes in and hits
the Bobo doll, then starts drawing some pictures and playing with

the dolls. She begins to develop all kinds of interesting dynamic themes such as stuffing the mother and father dolls down the toilet bowl; you are taking a flurry of notes. But as the interview goes on, the child moves away and becomes aloof, perhaps more passive. You feel at the end that you have lost a quickly made friend. While you should not interfere with the sequence of events in the opening interview, do note and learn from them.

To facilitate describing the quality of relatedness, it may be useful also to think of relatedness as evolving in the four general developmental levels or landmarks described in Chapter 1. Having these very general levels in the back of your mind may help facilitate even more detailed observations and descriptions of how the child is relating to you. These levels will be covered in more detail in the section on thematic organization and content.

The broad levels that one wants to consider start with whether the child engages at all. Early in life children learn both to attend and engage with their caregivers (often 'this is accomplished by 4 or 5 months of age). One wants, therefore, to observe first, as indicated earlier, how the child establishes a quality of connectedness and relatedness—gradually and slowly, quickly, or intermittently—and parallel with that, the degree of warmth and depth to that quality.

Added to the general quality of relatedness is how the child negotiates his relatedness with you. Does he organize his relatedness in an intentional way? Is there a sense that the child is negotiating a sense of relatedness with you, even through simple gestures? For example, the child who walks in and goes right for the toys, ignoring the clinician, is different from the child who looks at the clinician and, with a twinkle in his eye or a nod of his head, gestures an interest in the toys, and waits for a reciprocal gesture from the clinician that it's okay to open the cabinet or to pick up a game that might be on the floor. That simple gestural interchange suggests not only an aspect of communication, which will be discussed later, but also suggests an intentional, reciprocal, and, therefore, organized aspect to the relatedness. This child perceives relatedness as a two-way street where he provides and takes in information to negotiate the terms of the relationship.

Therefore, one begins to look for simple gestural cues—eye contact, simple pointing, simple sounds or vocalizations, facial expressions, motor gestures, and different subtle affect expressions. One notices here if the child initiates such gestures and if the child, in turn, responds to the clinician's counter-gesturing with a further gesture of his own. A simple "give me five," where a youngster offers the clinician "five," the clinician offers "five" back, and the youngster smiles, would be an example of the youngster taking some gestural initiative, the clinician responding, and the youngster, with an affect gesture, "closing a circle of communication." (A circle of communication, in terms of relating, is when the child initiates some aspect of relating, such as a smile, the clinician responds with a smile or a warm look back, and the child builds on the clinician's response with something in return, such as bringing a game over to see if the clinician will play with him or having the clinician look at a drawing, or pointing at a toy. When a circle is closed, it means that a child has initiated and then responded to some piece of relationship negotiation on the part of the clinician.)

When the child clearly evidences these first two elements of relatedness, engaging and then using simple gestures to negotiate the relationship, one can also observe if the child is capable of complex gestures to negotiate the relationship. Can the child begin using gestures to define and refine the quality of the relationship further, in terms of negotiating something about the meaning that the clinician has for the child, and the meaning that the child gives himself in the framework of the clinical setting? For example, the child who, when she can't quite open the door to the toy cabinet, comes over and points to the clinician and makes various sounds indicating "help me" is negotiating a complex meaning. An element of requesting help, perhaps even an element of dependency, is negotiated through the series of facial expressions, motor pointing, postural shifts, and grunts (even if the youngster is not talking, and many youngsters will obviously use words) to negotiate a complex meaning around dependency. At a later point in the interview, or even sometimes at an earlier point, the clinician may find himself negotiating limits with the child through a series of gestures where the clinician looks stern and frowns and puts his hand up like the corner policeman. Some youngsters will, after giving the clinician a mischievous grin indicating they are about to throw the ball at the clinician's head, stop with this limit-setting gesture on the clinician's part. Other children will throw caution to the wind, and the ball will come sailing by the clinician's eyes, if he is lucky and ducks fast enough. Here, one sees more complex gestures being used to negotiate meanings and the terms of the relationships. Will it be mutually respectful? Will it be chaotic and wild? Will it be evidenced by the clinician being helpful and supportive of the child's dependency needs? Or will it be characterized by the clinician ignoring the child's dependency needs? The clinician observes, in terms of this stage of relating, the degree to which complex meanings can be negotiated as part of the relationship. In other words, there is a difference between the child who engages the clinician, but seems satisfied to have the clinician look on warmly as the child plays (nothing much is happening interactively between them to negotiate the terms of the relationship), and the child who is related, but uses simple gestures and then more complex gestures to negotiate the meaning of that relationship. A whole drama can evolve between the clinician and the child around dependency, limit-setting and aggression, and curiosity, all without any words spoken. In the examples given above, I am deliberately portraying the child as nonverbal to illustrate how much can be learned before the child actually speaks or when the child is not actually speaking.

The next level in relating, however, does involve the child's ability to represent or symbolize experience, that is, to use words and make-believe play to negotiate further the quality of relating. Here, the verbal child has many options. She may ask the clinician for a particular toy, want to know what the clinician is going to do during this session, tell the clinician about worries and anxieties with the expectation that the clinician will be helpful, or share with the clinician her worries about what will happen in the clinical setting. In sharing her fears and anxieties, she may indicate a certain degree of trust or a certain degree of cautiousness about trying to define what's going to happen in the clinical interview. Alternatively, the child who develops pretend play sequences with hurricanes and disasters or with children getting injections may be indicating his expectations of this new relationship; or the child who has the dolls being fed and everyone being happy may be indicating a different set of expectations of the emerging relationship between the clinician and herself.

It is important to emphasize that this next level in relating, which, interestingly, occurs in normal development between about 18 months and 36 months, involves the child's using representations or symbols in both play and verbal communication (as well as sometimes in subtle spatial communications, such as building complicated towers or houses with passages in them).

The next level in negotiating the relationship concerns the child's not only using words or pretend play to convey his representational capacities, but also creating logical bridges between different islands of symbolic or representational communication. The child at this level doesn't just negotiate through a pretend drama where there are hurricanes or where the child doll is getting all kinds of goodies, but may, in a more reality-based way, begin negotiating the terms of the relationship with the clinician. "Can I do this?" or "Can I do that?" the child may say. "What will you do if I kick the ball into the wall?" the child may further ask. The child may also want to know if he and the clinician can play after the session is over because he enjoys the playroom so much (and seems to yearn for a little extra contact with other people). Every-thing from negotiations around bringing parents into the playroom, ending the session early, wanting to continue the session, wanting to know about the clinician's own children and family, to those around curiosity about where the clinician lives—in other words, any give-and-take that uses symbols or words in a logical interactive way, where there are logical bridges between one thought and another—suggests this more advanced level of negotiating rela-tionships.

Here, therefore, one gets a sense of the level of complexity and organizational status the child brings to negotiating relation-ships. Is he engaged? Does he use gestures in an intentional and reciprocal way? Does he use representation, symbols, or ideation to negotiate a relationship? Can he use ideas, symbols, or repre-sentations in a logical reality-based manner, as well as a pretend and fantasy-based manner?

As one is asking these broad developmental questions, one is also obviously looking for the particular contents and themes the child is interested in as part of relationships. Does she seem mostly concerned about dependency, having needs met? Does she seem mostly concerned about aggression and fear or injury and hurt? Does she seem mostly concerned about pleasure and excitement? Limit-setting can be negotiated with simple, stern looks or with complicated legalistic discussions of "Why can't I break your win-dows?" At each developmental level, from just the use of simple gestures to the use of more complicated ideas and symbols, these different relationship dramas can be played out.

In short, there are many possible patterns of relatedness. To determine relatedness, note your own subjective feelings; how the child relates to people in the waiting room; how he or she uses you during the interview; the spatial distance the child keeps as well as the verbal and eye contact he or she makes; and the child's emotional reaction to you versus his or her reaction to play mate-rials. Although you cannot generalize from such observations how the child forms all other relationships, you can note the obvious extremes—a detached, aloof, uninvolved child or a tense, hungry child who relates promiscuously—and the subtle gradations in be-tween.

Age expectations must also be taken into account. While all children optimally would be expected to develop an engaging sense of human involvement over time, with younger children the relat-edness may take on a more egocentric quality. By ages 4, 5, or 6, you may expect a capacity for more mutuality and even empathy.

AFFECTS AND ANXIETY

I have labeled the next category affects and anxiety. Here you want to observe both the specific emotions that get elaborated at the opening of the clinical interview and those that follow sequentially around particular activities. Again, you should begin observing the child in the waiting room and continue until you say good-bye and the child reengages with mother. Make at least a mental note of the different emotions the child shows. How does the child begin the session with you? What happens as he or she moves through the first third to the middle of the session, and then from the last third to saying good-bye? Follow the change in affect. For example: the child may come in showing apprehension and tentativeness; get warm and loving, and then competitive; show concern with issues of sibling jealousy and rivalry; and then express concern about separating from you toward the end of the interview. Here several specific feelings have been elaborated; in contrast, another youngster may show only one or two affects during the entire interview.

You want to be able to label all the different emotions you see in specified situations, and thus you may wish to take notes under headings for each of the categories. Some people feel that taking notes interferes with their involvement with the child and they prefer to rely on memory. In such instances, taking notes after the interview under systematic headings may prove useful. You may observe anger, competitiveness, envy, rage, compassion, empathy, affection, caring, emotional hunger, emotions expressing aggressive feelings, and emotions expressing passive yearnings.

The range and degrees of specific affects are very broad. In the aggressive domain, for example, one finds gradations from assertive behavior, to competitive behavior, to mildly aggressive behavior, to explosive and uncontrolled aggressive behavior. The same is true in the affectionate and caring domain, which ranges from promiscuous emotional hunger, to mild affection, to a sincere sense of warmth, to compassion, to the developmentally advanced emotion of empathy.

Children vary in the range of affect displayed. Some will show a wide range in the themes they develop. They may talk openly about warmth and pleasurable relationships, and indirectly about competition and envy. You will be able to see the dominant affects. Other children may be relatively quiet the whole time, displaying little emotion. There may be one isolated scene, such as the child's punching the Bobo doll and beanbag, which expresses the theme of loss.

In all cases you want to see how your observations fit in with what is to be expected of a child at his or her developmental stage. In a 3-year-old, for example, one does not expect as great a variety of differentiated affects as an 8-year-old would show. With a 3-year-old you can expect to see possessiveness, with some show of stubbornness and negativism. You can expect to see some capacity to share with you, and perhaps curiosity, pleasure, and excitement, but not more mature affects like empathy. By age 6 or 7, if you see negativism and aggression but no desire to explore, and no curiosity, assertiveness, or signs of empathy, you have to ask why the latter affects are missing.

You should observe and describe not only the range of affects but the richness and depth of affects. Are they superficial, as if the child is simply playacting or imitating someone? Or do they convey a sense of personal depth (i.e., you are able to empathize with the way the child is feeling)? Again, age expectations are important here. In a 3-year-old you expect some superficial imitation; by age 6 or 7 you expect to get a greater sense of the child's own personal affects.

You also want to get some picture of the age- and stage-appropriate stability of the affects. Is the child able to maintain an emotion throughout a reasonably lengthy period of communication with you? Or is the child emotionally labile, showing a wide range of affects (e.g., sadness, crying, elation, aggression) in a 2-minute period?

In considering affects, just as in considering relationships, it is helpful to have a developmental frame of reference in the back of your mind to facilitate the observation and understanding of specific affects and affect patterns. Are the affects, for example, part of trying to establish a sense of connectedness and relatedness—warmth, pleasure, a sense of intimacy and trust? If a sense of relatedness is affectively communicated, one might begin looking for how affects are used interactively, that is, to create intentional communication. Are certain affects used more in interaction than others? For example, which affects are part of two-way communication? The child may look longingly at you, establishing a hungry sense of relatedness, but when it comes to interactive signaling, he or she may deal mostly with themes of competition—"What's mine," "What's yours," "Who's going to win," and "Who's going to lose." In other words, against a foundation of warmth and security, the child interacts and negotiates themes of competitiveness and perhaps even power. Another child might engage and become close mostly through irritation—a provocative grin, rather than a warm longing or intimate feeling. This child may establish that response as his baseline way of relating, but actually choose not to negotiate or interact much with the provocativeness. In other words, he may not want your reaction to his gradual teasing, but just do it as a sort of background pattern. The negotiations may very well have to do with themes of hunger: "What's for me?" or "What can I take home with me?" Such a child may even want to put things in his pockets to make sure he doesn't lose them.

In addition to looking at the way the child engages, what affects are part of the engagement, and what affects are part of two-way communication, one also looks at the more complex forms of two-way communication in terms of what is being negotiated within a framework of meanings. How is the child dealing with or not dealing with broad themes of dependency, assertiveness, aggression, curiosity, or competition?

Just as one can observe the first three levels—the way the child engages, his initiation of simple interactions, his more complex interactions for negotiating important themes like dependency or limit-setting and aggression—one can also look at the fourth level, the way the child uses symbols or representations (words or pretend play) to communicate different affects. For example, the child may use gestures to communicate warmth and closeness—coming close, looking at you longingly, even a flirtatious glance or two—but not explore themes of closeness, warmth, or flirtatiousness in play with dolls or in any verbalizations. The verbalizations in the play may all have to do with competition and aggression. Conversely, the play themes may have to do with dolls hugging and kissing. The child may ask you if you like him and if he is your favorite person who comes in for therapy or play sessions. Yet while the child is asking this, the actual interactive style of the child might be oriented toward power struggles and competition, or even aggression.

Children may negotiate around certain affects (e.g., "who is the boss"). These affects are, therefore, interactive (e.g., gestural or representational). Other affects may be part of the quality of engagement, but they are never discussed, so to speak (e.g., the husband who expects to be cuddled but never gestures for or asks for "a hug" because he "doesn't know how").

Finally, one looks at the affects that the child can use in logical verbal interactions, or more elaborate pretend play where there are subplots all logically connected to one another. Do the child's more organized dramas have to do with envy, competition, excitement, anger, longing, neediness, or fear of separation? Similarly, in the more logical conversations of the child—the lawyer-to-lawyer conversations with lots of "buts," "becauses," and "ands and ifs" in them—what themes is the child negotiating? As one looks at affects, one looks at the affects that predominate, those that are less evident in the child's productions, and those that are not present at all. One also looks at which developmental level the child uses to organize different affects. Does the child seem to have access to representational forms or even highly differentiated representational forms (the logical bridging between different affects—"I'm mad because you came late to our session today"), or does he not (unable to represent his anger with words, he gives you angry glances)? Therefore, it is important to describe the range and type of affects and the developmental level at which the affects are organized.

You also want to notice the context in which the affects arise. A child who is engaging you in a certain style of relatedness may also be developing certain themes. Do the affects make sense in a thematic way, or are they inappropriate? Is the child showing joy and pleasure while cutting up the mother doll? Or does the child show compassion while burying a doll in the sand because it has just "died"? You want to note if the affects vary in relationship to the themes.

What we can call anxiety is related to the affects. Anxiety is not directly observed in the child, but it can be inferred from signs of distress or disruption. The best clue to points of anxiety is a sudden disruption in a developing theme, an ongoing style of relating, or a mannerism or gesture. During most play sessions, if you stay out of the child's way by not over-structuring the situation, you will see some disruption in activity when the child comes to an area that troubles her, and you will see what the disruption pathway is like for her in terms of personality structure. Did she show disorganized thinking and looseness in communication (equivalent to looseness of association in adults); did she lose impulse control, throwing or spilling things, or become clinging and want you to hold her?

For example, a child is playing with the mother and father dolls and develops the theme of the dolls fighting. She then darts to the other side of the room and begins behaving in a disorganized way, throwing things or messing up the floor with paint. You say to the girl, "That is not permitted because one rule of the playroom is that you cannot destroy things." She continues doing it, obviously disorganized and out of control. Finally she is about to spill the paint on your new suit and you have to restrain her. Here you have seen a profound disorganization occur.

Some children handle their distress by switching activities but carrying on the same theme in a less frightening mode. Again, let us say a child first develops the fighting theme with the mother and father dolls. Then, through a series of intermediaries, he shifts to drawing. He draws a cartoon with mother and father fighting and then draws some pictures of a less aggressive nature, showing that he wants to move into something less frightening. Here you see the ability to continue to work in a less frightening mode; the child has not given up entirely or become disorganized.

At first you will not know the nature of the anxiety, which may be fear of bodily damage, or of separation, or of some even earlier global anxiety. But you will know when there has been a disruption. At this point you just want to note its occurrence. When you go back over your notes and see the sequence of themes and affects, you will get some hints as to what caused the disruption.

You can learn a great deal simply by noting the sequence in a playroom session. The sequence of themes following a disruption may tell you what the child's fear centers on (e.g., bodily damage, world destruction, losing one's sense of self, losing the love of another person, abandonment). A sequence might run as follows: the child plays with the doll, darts over to the other side of the room and gets a gun, frantically shoots it at the dart board, and then goes back to the doll and starts shooting its arm off. Thus the child works a new theme—using the gun for violence—into the old drama. You have a picture of apprehension and anxiety; the theme seems temporarily broken, but then the child returns to it. He has armed himself but is still coming back into the "family" (the dolls). The sequence may suggest that he was concerned with some danger for which he felt a gun would be helpful. Therefore, one may hypothesize that the child is more concerned with physical, bodily harm than with separation or a more global loss.

By looking at disruptions in the child's play and communication from a developmental perspective, one may both look at the child's reaction to anxiety and determine if a child is, in fact, anxious. In a developmental framework, one can look for either a shift from a higher level to a lower level, a shift from a more adaptive pattern to a more maladaptive pattern at a given level, or a sudden narrowing of the thematic range. A shift from a higher level to a lower level does not always indicate anxiety. Sometimes, for example, in the excitement of play or simply in the relaxation of free expression, children may shift developmental levels in their mode of communication. However, this shift, coupled with other signs of anxiety, such as a change in facial expression, a sense of tension, an increase in motor discharge patterns, or an abrupt shift in content, will often indicate that anxiety is disrupting the child's play.

Consider the example of a child who is playing out themes in a highly representational, differentiated manner. He sets up the dollhouse with the hero dolls having a feast in their private castle. Suddenly, the heroes are attacked by the evil monster and his henchmen. The henchmen capture the good guys and tie them up to torture them. As the torture begins, the child shifts from organized make-believe play (or representational mode) and cause-and-effect logic ("The hero wasn't watching, therefore the monster was able to sneak up on him," etc.), to throwing the dolls around the room and pulling off the arms and legs with frantic activity, groaning and grunting, and hardly saying a word. Gradually, he seems less and less connected in an emotional sense to the clinician. Here, we see a child shifting from a representational differentiated mode to a prerepresentational behavior discharge mode, that is, he is behaving rather than representing experience. Furthermore, in the prerepresentational behavioral mode (the stage of intentional prerepresentational communication), he is not being organized, but being somewhat chaotic and even a little random. We therefore see a shift to an earlier developmental level and to a more maladaptive pattern in that earlier developmental level.

In a more subtle manner, the child may simply shift from a more differentiated representational mode to a less differentiated representational mode. For example, the dolls are having a tea party and the little girl asks the mommy doll to set the table. But the mommy doll says, "I'm busy now," or "I'm busy now and when I finish, I'm leaving." As the mommy doll introduces the theme of separation, the little girl stays representational but suddenly goes from a tea party with a logical interactive play theme to a tea party in a schoolroom, which then gets mixed up with a visit to the zoo and quickly changes to elephants and tigers all running around making silly noises. The scene keeps changing. The fragments of play are in a representational form—the little girl uses words and creates images in the pretend play rather than expressing herself through motor discharges—but they are fleeting images with fragments of meanings. When this kind of a shift occurs, we see a shift within a representational mode from a more differentiated, logical expression of meanings, even highly fantasized or pretend meanings, to one where the meanings, while still pretend, take on a more fragmented or less differentiated quality. Another way to think about this is that the pretend elaborations and verbal elaborations of the child lose their secondary process superstructure, and the structure of the communication, as well as the content, becomes primary process. In other words, the primary process aspects of communication can be viewed in terms of the content, as well as in terms of the structure or organization of the communication. Often, children who are developing fantasy themes will do so with secondary process elaboration. There is an organization to the drama. However, with such a shift, one may lose that and see primary process in both the content and the structure. This is a shift from the representational differentiated level to the less differentiated representational level.

The child who has a broad range of themes at a gestural or representational level, but then shifts to a narrow range of themes, may also be indicating some signs of anxiety. For example, the child who in his gestures is interacting in a warm and assertive, even empathic way (by how he respects the needs of the interviewer in terms of what things he can and cannot play with), but who shifts to an impersonal mode or just an aggressive or clinging mode, may be showing signs of anxiety, even though he stays within the behavioral mode. He is shifting from a broad-ranging flexible pattern to a more narrow and rigid pattern. The same implication would be drawn if this occurred at the representational level or the representational differentiated level.

Therefore, to discern anxiety, one can systematically examine the child's communication—play, verbalizations, gestures, or quality of engagement—and watch for shifts from a higher level to a lower level, shifts from an adaptive mode to a maladaptive mode at that level, or a narrowing of thematic range within a level.

When the child becomes anxious, it is often the interviewer's tendency to comfort him or her right away. The comforting is usually more subtle than putting one's arm around the child and saying, "Now, now, things will get better." For example, after seeing some acute anxiety, the interviewer may quickly begin structuring the activity by saying, "Why don't we try this," or, "Let's play checkers." A more sophisticated tack is to ask the child a question that diverts attention from the source of the anxiety to another area. We may say, "You know, you haven't told me about school yet. Tell me, how do you get along with the other kids at school?"

To be sure, if a child is becoming disorganized and cannot reorganize without help, you may need to move in a supportive way to help her reorganize her thinking and impulses. You can say something empathic, indicating that you understand her experience. Your remark should not focus on what stirred her up, e.g., "I can see that you don't like Mom and Dad fighting." The child who has played out such a fight scene and is already disorganized may not be able to deal with such a comment at that time. But if you say, "I know kids sometimes want to throw things and spill things," you are focusing on the child's tendency to get out of control rather than on what is scaring her. At the same time you are moving in, you are engaging and talking to the child, who will feel somewhat reassured. Such a course is much more reassuring than changing the topic. Also, after such a comment the child may be able to tell you about other instances when she was out of control.

The important point to note in the above example is that, for diagnostic purposes, it is necessary to observe the child's difficulty in coping before you take any action. You can be certain that whatever the child's behavior is in the playroom, it is worse at home. The child is not going to be destroyed if you remain silent for another 20 seconds. And the ability of a child to pull herself out without your help is such a vital diagnostic pointer that it is worth allowing the child to experience a little discomfort. Your whole treatment recommendation may hinge on such an observation, especially in cases where you are not sure whether the child's problems are predominantly character-ological or fall predominantly into the category of "borderline" psy-chopathology.

In summary, in addition to noting the child's specific range, richness, and depth of affects, it is equally important to observe their appropriateness in terms of the child's age and the themes being revealed. When play is disrupted by the emergence of troubling is-sues, you want to watch the child's reaction to the anxiety including shifts in developmental level, and the degree to which he can become reorganized without your help. Noting the themes that precede the disruption, as well as the sequence of those that follow it, should give you an indication of what the anxiety or fears relate to.

USE OF THE ENVIRONMENT

The next category covers the way a child uses the environ-ment—first the waiting room and then the playroom. Space in the office includes you as a human being, the inanimate objects such as the games and toys, and the space itself. What the child has is a multifaceted vehicle for communicating with you. Implicitly you have said, "Look, you have this room, these toys, and me. Now using these things, tell me something in the next 50 or 60 minutes." All children, even ones as young as 3 or 4 years, understand that the interview is a time for them to tell you something.

One of the first things you want to observe is whether the child can integrate the entire room. Such an ability will give you a picture of the degree to which the child can synthesize and integrate different elements in his or her own personality. The ideal way to use the space would be for the child to take it all in at the beginning, then move around and develop a few different areas, and finally synthesize the different areas. That is, a child may start with a view of the whole setup and develop a little story here, a little story there, and at the end you may see her beginning to weave together the little worlds she has developed for you.

For example, a child comes into the playroom apprehensively, goes into one corner and reveals some anxiety about the situation, and then begins exploring the playroom. She goes around and checks everything, then picks a few favorite areas, optimally interweaving them and relating them to one another. She takes a policeman doll from one part of the room, mother and father dolls from another part, and a lion from still another, and relates them to a theme of a policeman protecting the mother and father from the lion. This child not only develops a relatedness to her environment but tries to integrate its various elements.

In contrast, an obsessive or fearful child might move into one corner and stay there for the entire session. Another child may go all over the place impulsively, touching base with everything but never developing any of the areas. How the child initially approaches the space and how he eventually deals with it are useful data for you to record.

What I have been suggesting so far is that there is a great deal to observe in the interview that is quite independent of content: the child's physical neurological status, way of relating to you, overall mood, specific affects (including the moments of disruption), and use of space. Without knowing anything about content, if you provide vivid descriptions in all these categories, you will know a considerable amount about the developmental stage of the child and about what areas may be causing him difficulty.

As you consider the next categories—the depth, relevance, and sequence of the child's thematic organization and your own subjective reactions—you will develop further data about the child. It is important to highlight, however, that many interviews with children focus only on the thematic sequence and do not take advantage of the full range of observational data available.

THEMATIC DEVELOPMENT

The kinds of data included in the next category, thematic development, are in some respects subtler than those discussed so far. They involve analysis of the child's themes in terms of organization, richness and depth, age-appropriate relevance, and sequence. Here the word *themes* refers not only to the content of verbal communication but also to all the ways the child communicates—through gestures, drawing, playing, and other activities. Attention to thematic development will tell you a great deal about the child's characterological structure as well as the specific conflicts that the child may be experiencing at the time you are assessing him or her.

It will also yield clues to the appropriate course of treatment for the child. A child may come in with many conflicts and yet reveal a certain self-access that may permit easy, rapid movement in a treatment process. Other children may come with few manifest difficulties but show severe constrictions in the way they approach their own psychological lives. Observations along these lines will influence your choice of therapeutic strategies as well as your expectations of what will happen in the initial phases of therapy.

In considering thematic development, look first at the overall organization in terms of the presence or absence of logical links connecting the thematic elements. This process would be equivalent to observing the organization of thinking in an adult, but with important differences. In order to use such an approach with children, you must have an understanding of normal development and know what to expect at each age. Whereas with an adult you deal with one standard—a certain minimum capacity to organize thinking—with a child the standards vary according to age, and you must weigh the organization of themes against the age-appropriate standard.

For instance, if an adult reveals tangentiality in thinking and mild loosening of associations, you begin getting a picture of some fragility of the personality structure. With a child, however, the meaning of such signs depends on age. In a 4-year-old, we might not be surprised by the partial absence of logical links; in a 3½-year-old we would be even less surprised. In children of 6, 7, and 8, however, we expect a greater capacity to form logical bridges between thematic productions.

Moreover, even after long experience in working with children, making age-appropriate judgments is not always straightforward. For example, it is very hard to know what degree of thematic organization is to be expected in an Oedipal child who is just at the point of moving on from the fantasy-oriented thinking that characterizes the early years and becoming capable of reality-oriented thinking. This developmental point lies in that gray area between what Piaget calls preoperational thinking and concrete operational thinking. Often you see latency children who are still under the pressure of fantasy. You are not sure if they believe what they are saying or if there are logical links organizing what they are communicating. The following cases are examples of age-appropriate and age-inappropriate thematic organization.

Let us say that you have an 8-year-old boy who comes into the playroom and begins, appropriately enough, by punching a beanbag; he then takes a gun, starts shooting a target, and talks about angry feelings; then suddenly he falls to the floor, takes off his pants, and shows you his genitals. The absence of thematic linking here would raise a question in your mind about the organization of this child's thinking. It is the abrupt departure from one theme to another rather than the content itself that would startle you. An 8-year-old who wants to talk about his body after talking about aggression ordinarily would move through a series of steps. For example, he would talk about shooting in general, about shooting the dolls, and about how the dolls are hurt; then he would draw a picture of a body, and with empathic questioning by the therapist, he might talk about fears regarding his own body.

Consider another example. A 9-year-old boy comes into the interview room, makes good eye contact with the examiner, smiles, and asks if there are any games or toys to play with. The examiner asks what he has in mind, and the boy says, "Do you have a basketball? I like to play basketball." The examiner responds empathically—"Oh" is enough—and the child is off and running, telling you that he played basketball and made three baskets, etc.

As he talks about playing basketball, his emotional expression suddenly begins to get sad. When the interviewer wonders aloud about this change from glee and elation to a beginning look of sadness, the child says, "Well, I don't have enough friends to play with." He continues, "What a nice office you have here," and wonders if the therapist has children with whom he plays basketball. Then the child reflects on how often he has to play basketball by himself. Although he has a court near his house, his father will not play with him, nor will his brother, nor has he any friends that he can call on. Upon inquiry about his lack of friends, the boy describes a pattern of superficial relationships with schoolmates. Here we see an organized communication in the context of playing basketball, the theme being one of desire for greater emotional closeness and difficulty in achieving it comfortably. The theme is organized in that the elements emerge logically.

Let us continue this scenario—one in which we would have some question about the integrity of this child's organization of thinking. The child who has talked about playing basketball, and in this context about his loneliness, emotional hunger, desire for closeness, and lack of real friends, then wants to know if the interviewer will play basketball with him. When the interviewer asks how the child envisions this happening, he gleefully talks about their going out to the school yard and playing one-on-one.

Immediately following this remark, he says to the interviewer, "Can people die of heart attacks?" The interviewer wonders why that thought occurred to him and the child then says, "There was a car accident and people lost their arms and legs. Can robbers get into a building and steal?" When the interviewer asks for further elaboration, wondering what he means, the child stays on the topic of robbers getting into a building and stealing things. As the child talks about this, the interviewer finally gets the impression that the boy is talking about his concern over having something stolen from him.

In the foregoing example, we see an abrupt shift from the

interwoven themes of basketball, the wish for closeness, and feelings of loneliness and isolation, to themes of heart attack, physical injury, and things being stolen. A breakdown in thematic organization is signified by the absence of the connecting links that one would expect from a 9-year-old. Whereas the first segment reflects a relatively good capacity for thematic organization, in the second segment the child shows a breakdown in this capacity. If the child had not experienced this breakdown, you could have expected transitions concerning other sports, people getting hurt in sports, and the general issue of physical injury, eventually getting to the issue of being robbed. Such an alternative sequence represents an appropriate series for a 9-year-old. Through an explicit logic he would reach the same endpoint. The fantasy material concerning heart attacks, car accidents, and severed limbs would become elaborated less "from left field" and more with a series of thematic links or bridges.

The richness and depth of thematic development also deserve attention. Thematic organization reveals the degree to which a child has an age-appropriate capacity for reality testing and organized thinking or communicating. The richness and depth of thematic productions, on the other hand, should reveal the characterological or neurotic constrictions in the range of thought and affect available to the child. The child who is capable of developing rich, deep, age-appropriate themes is telling you that he or she has access to a rich, deep intrapersonal life. The child whose story is fragmented, superficial, or stereotyped, however, is telling you that consciousness of his or her intrapersonal life must be kept limited.

Soap operas and melodramas, with their shallow plots and cardboard characters, fail to convey a sense of richness and depth. By contrast, a novel is considered great to the extent that it attains that sense. In a similar fashion, a child's thematic development, as it unfolds in the clinical interview, may range from being superficial and fragmented to being complex and meaningful.

Let us say we have a 7-year-old girl whose early development was troubled and whose Oedipal phase was poorly negotiated. Only partial closure was achieved at the expense of a great deal of inhibition around various sectors of the personality, such as anger, assertion, and even empathy or concern. In watching this child, you may see a lot of scattered associations. She may go for the doll and then go play with the gun, then start to draw a house. What will be notable is that you will not see any development of themes. In other words, there will be no unfolding of a story. Now even though a child, unlike an adult, does not tell you an organized story with feeling, if you sit with a child and do not interfere with what she does, a story of one kind or another will surely unfold.

A child such as this 7-year-old, who can portray only shallow bits and pieces of a drama, may be demonstrating many developmental blockages. The girl wants to tell more about her angry feelings, yet that leads to anxiety; she wants to tell more about some caring feelings, but that leads to anxiety; she wants to tell more about fears that she experiences (all indirectly, to be sure), and that way is blocked. Thus you may see a scatter of thematic material at a superficial level.

Admittedly, this lack of depth is hard to diagnose. It cannot be diagnosed simply by noting that the child moves to many different parts of the room or uses many different materials. Even though a child may behave in an active and even anxious way during the session, you can often see progression in the development of a theme. You have to ask, What kind of understanding did I get? How deep and rich was the material that this child was able to portray for me? These reflections will give you a picture of the degree of potential restrictions.

Here, too, in assessing the richness and depth of thematic development, you need to know the age-appropriate expectations. For example, from a latency child of 7½ or 8 you should expect some constricted thematic development, at least in the first diagnostic playroom interview, because of the nature of the defenses developed during latency. In such children you often see support of the repression that follows the Oedipal phase, with the use of reaction formations, and sometimes even the beginning of some isolation of affects. You may expect that latency children will fend you off, protecting their turf. However, the way in which they protect their turf may have a certain richness and depth to it. While taking the stand, "I'm not going to tell you everything you want to know and don't ask me too many personal questions at this time," they may yet be giving you a sense of their flexibility.

An Oedipal child, on the other hand, is usually capable of rich elaboration of fantasy. Some people think the Oedipal stage is the most creative time in one's life because of the abundant availability of thematic material. If you see a 5-year-old who is shallow and constricted you would certainly have questions. As you work with 5-year-olds, you will readily see the ease with which they get into a great variety of material; a lack of such easy variety may be a signal that there are developmental interferences or conflicts.

For example, a 5-year-old boy may come in, look at you, make meaningful eye contact, sit down, and ask, "What am I supposed to do?" When you ask him what his guess is, he may say, "Oh, I'm supposed to talk about my worries and fears." He spots a gun over in the corner of the room and asks, "Can I play with that?" After the interviewer nods affirmatively, the boy goes over and picks up the gun. He then begins a game of shooting the mother doll and the father doll, as well as going "bang, bang" at the interviewer.

Following the game of shooting, he takes the baby doll and puts it in a safe place in the corner of the room without comment. The interviewer wonders out loud, "Gee, you are putting the baby doll over in that corner of the room." The child replies, "Yes, I want to make sure it is safe." The interviewer says, "You mean from all the shooting?" The boy replies, "I don't want it to be hurt." The interviewer says, "How's that?" and the little boy goes over and gets the doctor kit out and begins taking care of the baby doll, bandaging it and making sure it is all right. He explains that the doll got caught in the cross fire, had its legs and arms cut off, and had an injury to its nose. In talking about the doll being hurt, he conveys some pretended sadness and then decides, "I'm going to get the robbers who did that."

He then sets up a game where he is a policeman shooting it out with the bad guys. Following this, he talks about how people have to be careful about bad guys who "steal things." The therapist empathically says, "Yes, I can understand how one could be concerned about controlling those bad guys who steal things." At this, the boy elaborates on all the things that bad guys would want to steal—his television set, his money, and more, finally getting to his baby brother. As the interview progresses, he continues to develop the themes of bad guys stealing, and policemen and good guys protecting.

Then the child becomes curious about what is going on behind the doors of the interview room. The interviewer asks what he thinks is going on. He says, "I don't know," and then goes over to the dolls and develops a complicated interaction where the mother and father doll are fistfighting and then go into the bathroom together. This sequence continues as he develops more themes related to what mother and father do together and what they do in the bathroom.

The foregoing example shows a child capable of developing an organized, rich, deep drama. His story contains violence and protection (e.g., robbers and cops), and it reveals the various sides of his own wishes: to take things, to rob, and to protect the family against such wishes and impulses. He then reflects on a theme related to his interests in robbing and protecting, that is, what goes on behind closed doors. His story shows his curiosity about his parents, and what they do in the bathroom and other rooms that are closed off to him. Here is an example of the development of themes (which are also appropriate for a child of this age) that gets richer and deeper as the interview goes along.

Consider a contrasting illustration. A 5-year-old boy comes

in and starts the interview in the same way as the first child: he goes after the gun and shoots it, and then sees the Bobo doll in the corner and starts punching it. The boy shoots and punches the Bobo for the next 15 minutes. The interviewer comments, "Gee, you really enjoy shooting and punching the Bobo." The boy looks at the interviewer as though to nod in agreement and continues the shooting and punching. Finally tired of the Bobo, the child goes around and shoots up the various dolls and the room in general. The interviewer again comments on the boy's desire to shoot, the child again gives a look to the interviewer indicating agreement and continues shooting.

The child sees a ball and asks the interviewer to play catch with him. They begin to throw the ball back and forth. The interviewer tries a number of times to have the child verbalize or develop in a richer way what might be on his mind, but the child sticks to alternating between throwing a ball and shooting the gun at the Bobo and other targets. Throughout this period, the boy makes good eye contact and seems reasonably affable. He is willing to come physically close to the interviewer. Near the end of the interview, desperate to get some more material, the interviewer suggests drawing, and the child draws a picture of a gun shooting a house. He then draws a picture of a child throwing a ball.

Here we have an example of a child who clearly shows that the theme of aggression (hitting and shooting) is on his mind, but we could say that there is very little richness or depth to the theme. What develops in the first few minutes of the interview is not further developed; rather, there is a repetitive quality to the child's communications, or thematic development, in contrast to the earlier example of ever-increasing richness and depth.

As mentioned earlier, you would not necessarily expect the same type of thematic depth and richness in an 8½-year-old as you would in a 5-year-old. An 8- or 9-year-old's personality ordinarily tends to be a little more rigid and stereotyped. Indeed, the competent latency-age child may successfully defend against many interesting fantasies. For example, an 8-year-old girl may come into the interview room and say, "I don't know why I am here. I haven't much to talk about." Then she may show some interest in playing checkers with the interviewer. There may be some discussion of the rules of the game that the child brings up—she wants to be sure that "we both understand in advance." As the rules of the game are elaborated, we see the child go into great detail, making sure that neither she nor the interviewer cheats. The interviewer inquires further about the importance of rules in connection with cheating. The girl then describes in elaborate detail the various ways one can cheat in playing different games. She talks about how friends at school sometimes cheat and says, "I have to be the one who is careful and not let them get away with it." The theme of cheating is also elaborated in terms of her 5-year-old brother, who, she says, "likes to take advantage of me sometimes. He steals my things and gets into my games. I have to be careful of him." This theme then gets developed in terms of other family members. The girl goes on to say that she is not so sure whether her father is a person who plays by the rules or not. Then quickly she says, "I know my father is a person who knows the rules and plays by the rules."

This interview starts off with typical latency-age defenses, but develops thematic richness and depth even though the child is at an age at which fantasy life is thought to be more restricted along the dimension of control. The example demonstrates that latency children are as capable of developing rich, deep themes as are Oedipal children, except that the direct access of the latency child to the underlying fantasy may be less facile. The healthy latency child may develop a rich, deep theme around the desire for control and regulation and how he or she has to contend with "those forces and people" who do not have similar inclinations.

Contrast the above example with a 9½-year-old girl who comes into the interview room and, instead of developing a rich, deep theme around rules and regulations stemming from a game of checkers, begins to play checkers, then switches to playing chess, and then switches to playing Monopoly, talking very little during any of these activities. This child, although concerned with rules, is more concerned with winning. She merely talks about the rules per se, sticking very much to the concrete details. There is almost no spontaneous elaboration about the implications of what she is doing. When she shows concern about "making the right moves" so that she will not lose her checkers, and the interviewer comments empathically that it's understandable that someone would want to make sure she did not lose any checkers, the child does not take off from this and talk about the theme of loss but continues talking about the checkers, never elaborating beyond the concrete level of the game. This girl, in contrast to the child in the above example, stays at a fairly superficial, fixed, and stereotyped level.

As indicated, the range and depth of thematic development provide a good initial picture of certain structural aspects of a child's internal life. The next subcategory, thematic sequence, is a source of clues to the nature of the child's particular concerns. Up to now, we have not talked about the content of the issues troubling a child. We have been discussing the form and structure of the personality—the theater in which the drama is portrayed. To see the drama, you must pay attention to the sequence of thematic productions. The drama's content may be murky, the issues disguised, but close examination of the sequence of themes will clarify what lies at the core—fear of closeness or separation, concern with various kinds of danger to one's body, rivalry with a younger sibling, etc.

For example, take a 6-year-old girl who takes all the family dolls and dramatically stuffs them into the toilet bowl. Then she gets scared and drops this play, thereby disrupting the thematic progress. She becomes hyperactive and starts punching the Bobo in a frenzied way. Following that, she calms down on her own and draws a family scene in which she is next to her father and her mother is far away. Then she smiles.

What does such a sequence suggest? She starts out with a theme of stuffing everyone down the toilet, from which you could hypothesize that she has either a wish to stuff or a fear that she will be stuffed down. Then there is anxiety and frenzied activity sufficient to create difficulty in getting her attention for a while, showing that probably the aggressive scene frightened her. Then she demonstrates that she is able to reorganize her capacity to communicate by calmly drawing a picture of the family, presumably the way she would like it to be, with her next to father. From this sequence, we can hypothesize concerns with overcrowding (i.e., in the toilet bowl) in the family, aggression (some questions about what goes on in the bathroom), and a wish to be close to father in the family structure. Her ability to reorganize and return to the theme of family structure, reflecting her own (smiling) wish, shows her capacity for integration.

Consider the example of a latency-age boy. He is talking about school and says that the kids poke fun at him and that the teacher is not treating him fairly or being protective. The next theme concerns a brother or sister who gets more attention than he does at home. Then he stops talking to you and finds a gun to play with or starts shooting darts. After that he gets curious as to why he is there with you and wants to know something about you. You ask him what he has been told or what he thinks. He responds that you are a doctor who helps kids and you seem nice. You then comment that, in here, he feels that maybe he does not have to worry that someone will take advantage of him. In other words, via the above sequence of thematic development, this child is telling you that the world is unfair and that he hopes you are different but he is not sure. He wants you to reassure him.

Another child comes in placidly, sits down, and gives you a look that says, "Okay, now entertain me." You wait a few minutes and then comment that it seems he just wants to sit and watch for a while, and you wonder what is going through his mind. That very passive child may eventually begin drawing explosions and cars crashing into one another. He may be too frightened to smash up the toy cars or take the toy gun and start shooting. Such a sequence yields a picture of a passive child with fears of explosive aggression.

The thematic sequence tells you not only what the core issues are but how they relate to one another. For example, a boy begins by shooting the gun and then looks scared; he takes a girl doll and looks under the dress, then throws it down. The child announces that he is "the strongest of all" and you comment that he sounds as if he is stronger than everyone else. He says, "Yes, I am stronger than my little brother. I can beat him up. I can even beat up my mother and father." Here you see a child who starts off with aggression, shows curiosity about the anatomy of girl dolls, and then makes himself powerful in order to deal with the fears and anxiety surrounding this aggression (i.e., a counterphobic style).

In the next sequence you may see this child becoming frantic, moving around the room and throwing things. You make a comment that he seems to be moving quickly and wants to throw everything around. Sometimes such a child then settles down and begins drawing pictures that express themes of yearning and early dependency. To return to the above example, once this child gets used to you and to the playroom, he may begin moving closer to you, wanting to involve you in the play. You get a subjective feeling of a strong yearning for close contact with someone. You may later sense, through drawings or other play, some feelings of emptiness. In summary, if you see aggression followed by dependency and yearning, you will have strong evidence that there is a significant relationship among these three issues.

Take one of the earlier examples, in which the child comes in, takes the gun, starts shooting, and then puts the baby doll in a safe place and begins doctoring and bandaging it. He then shows curiosity about what is going on behind the playroom door and develops a family drama about what his parents do in the bathroom and behind closed doors. This sequence gives a good picture of the nature of his concerns. It suggests, first, that he is concerned with his angry wishes, which are in conflict with his protective and caring wishes, and second, his curiosity about what his parents are doing behind closed doors. If, after talking about his parents, he begins talking about children getting sick and a cold he had the other day, and then wonders about going to the hospital and recalls his last visit to the doctor, we may see that his curiosity is also associated with fear of physical injury. His interest in what goes on behind closed doors and what goes on in the bathroom may be associated with fear about what can happen to him. From this example, we see how the thematic sequence gives us a ready and clearly interpretable picture of how concerns are related to each other in a child's mind.

Consider another example. A 7-year-old girl comes into the room and goes to the dollhouse, where she begins playing with the mother doll. She rounds up the family of dolls and uses a crayon to color over the dolls' faces. She then tries to detach the head of one of the dolls; not succeeding, she tries another doll and is able to rip off the head. There is a gleeful, somewhat eerie expression on her face; her eyes light up and she immediately grabs a ball and throws it against the wall, jumping around in a disorganized fashion. She runs over to the other side of the room and says she wants to play catch. She starts throwing the ball against the wall, narrowly missing some of the interviewer's favorite decorations. She continues this behavior, becoming more disorganized and fragmented. The interviewer comments on this behavior, which only makes it worse. Finally, the interviewer interrupts and suggests that they put the feelings into words rather than actions. When this tactic does not work, the interviewer has to go over and take away the ball lest all the furniture be broken.

This sequence suggests something fundamentally different than those discussed earlier. Here the girl shows her concern with aggressive themes by pulling off the head of a family member, but then she becomes disorganized and chaotic and cannot reorganize herself. She cannot return to the thematic area. We see aggression followed by disorganization. This not only tells us something about the child's concerns, but also suggests that she is unable to handle these concerns, that they tend to disorganize her. She is not able to shift into a protective or caring mode, to change the theme on her own, or to demonstrate other maneuvers that would help her to deal with her frightening aggressive impulses. She was able to move away from the anxiety-laden situation only by abandoning herself to a general disorganization and impulsivity. Even though impulsivity in latency-age girls is less frequent than in boys of the same age, when it exists, it will emerge readily in the thematic sequence if the interviewer doesn't prematurely structure the situation.

As you learn to follow the sequence carefully, you will also be able to identify the developmental levels of the core conflicts. In other words, the dependency or the anger can exist at many levels. By examining the sequence closely, you will get some hunches as to whether the child's fears are age-appropriate.

For example, a 5-year-old may express an interest in your person that focuses on "what's hidden under your clothes," an age-appropriate curiosity. You may observe conflicts about this curiosity in the form of fear of body parts falling off (e.g., arms and legs of dolls falling off). In contrast, this same 5-year-old may show an interest in your person around themes of emotional hunger or basic security together with fears of global destruction and disorganization. Such themes are representative of developmentally earlier concerns.

As indicated, the thematic sequence provides clues about the nature of the child's concerns. The interviewer's goal is to follow the sequence of the child's thematic productions with minimal interference. Any comments should facilitate movement in the direction the child has chosen. They should *not* take the child in a new direction. The child's associations, one following another, will tell you his or her story better than any responses to your directions.

As discussed earlier in this chapter, you should note the sequences of events in the other categories as well (e.g., the sequence of the quality of relatedness to you, the sequence of the affects). When you combine your observations on the sequences of the content, the relatedness, and the affects, you have the material you need to make hypotheses about the child's conflicts. For example, from looking at the symmetry between the sequences of content and affect you can begin to get clues about the personality structure of a child. From the thematic development of an 8-year-old with an integrated ego structure, you may expect to learn something about the child's internal life and concerns; then ask yourself if these concerns are symmetrical to and integrated with the child's affects. The affects that emerge may point to anxiety and tensions around the disturbing issues. You might hypothesize, for example, that the child is having some conflicts within the context of a basically intact ego structure.

As with the other categories, it is useful to observe the child's organization of his communication and its content from a developmental perspective. While this developmental perspective has been implied throughout this discussion on thematic organization and development, it is especially valuable for the clinician to have a systematic model in the back of his or her mind. This will make it easier to think about both the organization of the child's thematic communication and its specific content. In a broad sense, the clinician wants to be coming at this material from the ground up, asking first, "Is the child able to be attentive and related while communicating with me?" In other words, is the child aloof and playing on his own, mechanical, cold, or withdrawn? Or is there a sense of warmth and connectedness as he plays out his make-believe drama or simply uses gestures to communicate wants and desires? Along with the quality of relatedness, how focused and attentive is he? The clinician asks, "Can he focus on me as he talks to me, or does he talk to me in fleeting bits and pieces as he strolls around the room looking at the pictures or out the window, fiddling with a glass, playing with the pillows?"

Secondly, as the child is communicating, one wants to understand how much he can organize simple gestures in an intentional manner. How does he come into the room and greet the clinician? Is there eye contact, a smile, or a grin? Or is there a look of fear and apprehension? Can the interviewer get a sense of the child's inclinations from his gestures, or does the child appear flat, chaotic, or random in his use of gestures? If the simple gestures are working for the child—the looking, pointing, body posture, a smile, a frown, or a look of interest, curiosity, or excitement—how does the child deal with his more complex gestures, those having to do with negotiating more complex communication patterns with the interviewer? For example, how does the child define his space? Does he use gestures to invite the interviewer to be very close, to come down on the floor with him and play almost nose-to-nose? Or, with his body posture and the way he looks at the interviewer and uses vocal tone and cadence, does he give the message, "Stay away. Give me distance. Give me lots of space"? How does he deal with limits in the room? Does he respond to the interviewer's complex gestures with limits when the interviewer looks concerned or makes an arm movement to indicate, "Not that toy," or "Don't throw that toy," or "Let's get organized here. We have to clean up"? Body posture, gesture, and facial expression, as well as words, communicate these messages. How does the youngster organize these signals, and deal with them? How does the child use gestures to communicate mutual respect, or even mutual pride and admiration, to the interviewer? Do they exchange looks of pleasure and pride? Do they use their body posture, arm and leg movements, and affect cues to communicate areas of mutual respect, pride, and pleasure? Or are these emotional themes not part of the organized gestural system?

It is very useful for the interviewer to determine, in a systematic way, both how well the child uses simple gestures for greeting, departures, or acknowledgment of another person, and how well the child uses complex gestures to negotiate important interpersonal, prerepresentational meanings (dependency, aggression and its limits, acceptance and pride, admiration, disapproval, rejection, annoyance, empathy for the other person's uniqueness, etc.). As described earlier, all of these characteristics can be communicated with gestures as well as with words. While often words and gestures will be used simultaneously, the clinician wants to make an independent judgment about the gestural part of this system before focusing exclusively on the child's verbal communications (if the child is a verbal child).

Therefore, at the prerepresentational or preverbal level, the clinician is looking at how the child communicates and organizes themes in terms of relatedness; the depth, warmth, and quality of intimacy; the way the child reengages; the child's attentiveness and focus; the child's use of simple gestures; and the child's use of complicated gestures. The clinician is also looking at how these early levels of communication are employed around different themes. What can the child use complex gestures for? Only for warmth and closeness, but not for negotiating aggression or limits? Or for both? Only for mutual respect and admiration, but not for closeness or limits? Or for all three? In other words, is the child at this gestural level, and if so, can the child use it with all the age-appropriate themes he is concerned about?

At the next level, the clinician looks at the child's ability to use representations or ideas in pretend play or in the intentional use of words. "Give me that," "I'm sad," or "I'm happy" are all intentional uses of words, as opposed to descriptive uses such as "That's a lamp" or "That's a chair." Pretend play, where the animals are having a tea party, hugging, or fighting, communicates emotional themes. Both of these are signs that the child is representational.

The clinician then asks whether the child is representational in the way he plays out or communicates his themes, and if the child is representational, the clinician next asks which themes the child brings into the representational or symbolic mode. In other words, does the child, when he is angry, use only gestures and behavior to communicate his anger, such as angry glances or actually biting and hitting, or is the child able to elevate aggression to the representational mode where he can create scenes of soldiers or animals fighting? Or, can he use words and say things like, "Me mad?" There is a difference between the prerepresentational organization of anger and the representational organization of anger. Similarly, with dependency, do the dolls hug? Does the child say, "Me like you," or "Me love you," or "Can I come back?" Or does he deal with dependency only with actual hugs or clinging or even grabbing possessions and wanting to take them home? Again, is the behavioral mode used or has the child advanced to representational elaboration in dealing with these basic themes of life? If the representational mode has been reached, what themes can it accommodate? Does it accommodate all the themes that the child is likely to be interested in, or only some of these themes? Is it broad and rich, or narrow and constricted?

Next, the clinician looks at the degree to which the child has progressed beyond the simple representational mode to the more differentiated representational mode. The child not only represents themes in pretend play and in intentional language, but now creates logical links to bridge one representational element with another. The dolls are fighting *because* they are mad at each other, *because* one doll took the favorite food of another doll. Here we see two "becauses" linking up the different elements. Does the child argue with the therapist? "Last week you promised to play checkers with me today. You forgot, didn't you?" As the therapist explains that he never made the promise, the child says, "Remember, halfway in the session, right after you took your telephone call, which I didn't like by the way, you made a promise to make it up to me." The clinician, feeling guilty, says, "Oh, yes. I think I remember." Here we see a logical, reality-based child using words in a highly intentional and organized manner, showing differentiated thinking in a disagreement with the clinician about the activity of the day. Whether it is the interlocking of complex themes—the tea party evolves into dinner, mommy and daddy argue over what is for dessert—or whether it's a lawyer-to-lawyer conversation about the rules of the playroom, the representationally differentiated child will have logical links connecting his themes.

Besides looking for logical links, one also looks at how the child applies these logical links to a broad range of themes. Is the child's range broad or narrow? Does she bring in dependency but not aggression, or only aggression but not dependency? Curiosity, but not dependency and pleasure? Which particular themes have exposure or access to this highly differentiated representational mode?

One also looks at the child's ability to go even beyond representationally differentiated modes of communication and mobilize extended representational systems and multiple extended representational systems as seen in latency-age children. In other words, can the child now build logic upon logic and see the relative relationships, the shadings and gray areas, between different themes? Can the child construct a complex logical matrix for her pretend or fantasy elaborations or her reality-based concerns? For example, the full-latency child with extended representational systems or multiple extended representational systems will derive from her basic concerns themes that are connected to each other logically. The animals might be angry at each other, but then because they have a common goal of defending against the enemy, they decide to be nice to each other and make peace. But within that peace treaty they distrust each other. To some degree, they are always watching what the others are doing. As long as they have the common enemy, they are willing to work together. As they work together, they get to like each other a little bit better and trust each other even a little bit more. An inkling of distrust exists, but the trust is growing. By the end of the enterprise, the common defense of their castles leads them to be comrades in arms, realizing that sometime in the future they may be enemies again, but for now they are going to have a party and celebrate their victory. The child is able to reflect that you can compete with someone and still be friends with that individual, particularly when there is a common enemy on the outside. This type of highly complex drama, with shades of gray (competition and aggression in a framework of collaboration) would not be possible for a 4-year-old or a 5-year-old. It is quite possible for a bright 7-year-old, but more likely for a 9- to 10-year-old, to mobilize this kind of complicated, logical infrastructure for his pretend dramas. It shows the stages of representational differentiation, extended representational systems, and multiple extended representational systems. This type of play signifies a high level of organization in the child's communications.

To use this framework clinically, one pictures first which developmental level a child has more or less attained in his communicative capacities. This tells you something about the thematic organization. One then pictures the different themes of emotional life. One way of doing this is to think of the following themes: dependency and closeness; pleasure, excitement, and sexuality; assertiveness, curiosity, competition, anger, and aggression; self-limit-setting; and empathy and more mature forms of love. These themes encompass much of the emotional human drama.

With the above themes, also consider their flip sides: part of dependency includes separation anxiety; part of aggression includes fears and worries about aggression. One can slice the emotional pie in different ways. But it is important to have a systematic way of categorizing the different emotional themes of life and then to superimpose these emotional themes on the developmental levels. In other words, one now looks at the degree to which a developmental level can organize certain themes and not organize others. For example, how does a child deal with dependency and closeness? Does he use highly differentiated extended representational capacities, or just gestures? Does he become aloof and distant, not even engaging and attending when he is dealing with themes of dependency, avoiding them almost entirely? For each emotional theme, one can see the developmental level used to communicate that particular concern, or not to communicate that particular concern, i.e., when the child seems to want to run away from it. It should be pointed out, however, that in this framework, the child invariably communicates about all these emotional themes in one way or another. In this framework, even disengagement and aloofness are ways of communicating.

For example, the next natural step in the pretend play is a sequence about closeness or concern about separation, and, at this point, the child becomes aloof, distant, and begins perseverating by opening and closing a little play door in a mechanical manner. Such a shift may be the child's way of indicating his particular concerns about closeness, dependency, and separation. When it comes to these concerns, he becomes aloof or uninvolved with the people on whom he feels most dependent.

In addition to looking at the organizational level achieved, one also looks, as suggested before, at the sequence of themes. As indicated earlier, if the child always follows aggression with disengagement or disorganization, one senses that aggression is conflictual and anxiety-provoking. If he always follows aggression with fear of injury and disorganization, one gets a sense of both sides of the conflict. On the other hand, if he always follows a desire for closeness with separation scenes and anxiety and either a shift to a lower developmental level or a maladaptive pattern at the existing developmental level, one gets a different sense of the two sides of the conflict. A more complex fantasy may emerge, with conflictual elements and nonconflictual elements. The sequence of the child's themes in the play may show that dependency is followed by aggression, then fears of injury, withdrawal, and finally aloofness. Here, one sees a more complex drama with a number of elements to it. It is as though the child is saying, "I want to be close, but when I come close, there is a lot of anger in relationships." (The child, at this point, is not making it clear whether this is his own or someone else's anger, or perhaps even a combination of both.) Then the child becomes concerned with injury and decides to withdraw from relationships as a safety precaution. The sequence, therefore, reveals the way in which the child sees an aspect of his world.

It is especially important to look at the different developmental levels the child brings to bear in organizing his fantasy. Consider the child mentioned above: He seeks out dependency at a representational level, then plays out themes of aggression, and then has people being hurt (also at a representational level). Then let's say that rather than having the dolls become aloof and go back to their own house (playing out disengagement at the representational level), he instead shifts and actually becomes aloof and withdrawn himself. The child is shifting from the representational level to the two prerepresentational levels concerning gestures and engagement as he intermittently becomes aloof after the themes of aggression and injury emerge. He is quite different from a child who plays out the theme of disengagement by having each of the dolls go back to its own home and be alone. An even more typical example is the child who starts with the dolls fighting and soon shifts from the "pretend" level to jumping on or throwing a ball at the clinician. It is easy to fool oneself and think this is still "pretend." As the clinician is ducking, it would be wise for him or her to recognize that the child has shifted to the level of behavioral discharge.

The child who plays his themes out at the representational

level is organizing all of his psychological life at the representational level (i.e., the child can express that desire to be alone either through words or pretend play while remaining engaged). The child who actually becomes aloof and withdraws is quite different. Picture these two children as adults: One, when he has an argument with his wife, is able to say, "I feel so lonely after we fight. I wish we could remain close somehow." The other needs to actually leave the room and go off by himself and maybe not talk to his spouse for a few days. Therefore, the developmental level and content of themes must be viewed together. When the developmental level is age-appropriate, there is another aspect of thematic communication that is important.

An aspect of thematic development that I have emphasized throughout this discussion is the assessment of age-appropriate relevance. Is the child concerned with the kinds of issues that you would expect, given your understanding of his or her background in terms of subculture, religion, and other relevant aspects? Is the child dealing with issues that seem above or below the age-appropriate level? Such questions will shed light on the content of the conflicts and how the child deals with them. The 13-year-old boy who talks about things that you expect to hear from a 7-year-old indicates his fear of entering adolescence and the degree of that fear. You frequently see early adolescents who are lingering in latency and, similarly, latency children who are behaving much more like Oedipal youngsters. For example, a 6-year-old boy may give you glimpses of 6-year-old behavior with competitive, assertive, or phallic themes. The child also displays negativistic belligerence and defiance, saying, "I won't do anything you want me to." He sits in the middle of the room and wants to be king of the place, ordering the therapist around. This boy is curious about things in the room, wants to know what is behind the doors, builds a few towers, but then quickly goes back to being negativistic and bossy, throwing things down and demanding that the therapist pick them up for him. Here we see movement between Oedipal themes and anal, pre-Oedipal ones. This kind of movement indicates that, although the child is working in the age-appropriate sphere, he must be frightened because he keeps retreating to earlier defensive positions.

On the other hand, the earlier example of the 5-year-old who starts shooting and then puts a baby doll in a safe place and begins bandaging it was rather typical of an Oedipal-age child. In his concerns—namely, competitive feelings toward a sibling, conflicts about aggressive and protective feelings, interest in his parents' bathroom and bedroom, and worries about the physical integrity of his own body—he is showing a number of age- and phase-appropriate Oedipal problems.

In summary, the aspects of thematic development discussed here include thematic organization, which focuses on how thematic elements are connected; the themes' richness and depth, which concern the degree to which a child can develop a story before encountering restrictions or blocks that impede the unfolding of the story; thematic sequence, which contains clues to the child's concerns and core issues as well as to the kinds of defenses the child used against the concerns; and the themes' age-appropriate relevance, which signals both the age level from which some of the child's conflicts derive and how the child handles the conflicts. Observations of these thematic elements will allow you to develop hypotheses about the child's characterological structure and central fears and conflicts.

SUBJECTIVE REACTIONS

The final category of observation concerns your own subjective reactions. There are two aspects to consider: the general feelings that the child evoked in you and your fantasies during the interview. When you examine your reaction at the end of the interview, you want to know how the child made you feel—drained, elated, angry, frustrated, or what? Do you feel as though you conducted the interview poorly? Do you feel depressed about your own performance? Or do you feel as though you are the best diagnostician in the world?

For example, little girls sometimes tell a male interviewer everything he wants to know, making him feel masterful. After such a session you feel terrific, as if you had hardly even been working. The fact that you are feeling so great with this young girl may be a clue to the fact that she is dealing with significant Oedipal issues. On the other hand, if a male therapist is with a young boy who is being warm rather than competitive, and who makes the therapist feel good, the therapist's feelings may be a sign that the child is coping with some negative Oedipal issues affecting defensive structures.

Be very honest with yourself. What you are feeling is in some way related to the child and is separate from your own level of experience or competence. You will find that, no matter how experienced or inexperienced you are, with certain children you will feel competent and talented whereas with others you will feel inept and inadequate, as if you were tripping over yourself all the time. Such differences in your own reaction are significant: other things being equal, children who make you feel frustrated are quite different from children who make you feel good.

In addition to examining your general reaction, you also want to look at the sequence of specific fantasies that occur to you during the course of the diagnostic. If anything unusual comes to mind (e.g., highly personal memories or images), or if you find yourself not listening for a moment or two while attending your private associations, such a reaction may reflect your unique transference to this child. Later on, when you have time to reflect, discover what idiosyncrasy of yours started this line of thought. Then ask yourself why this thought came to you at this particular point in the interview. Regardless of what motivated this thought—be it hostility, exhibitionism, or whatever—use the information to understand why the child stimulated this response in you.

For example, too often we merely feel guilty if we find we have stopped listening. But if you feel yourself getting bored or sleepy, you should ask yourself, What is this child doing that elicits this reaction in me? The effect is immediately to make you more vigilant as you seek some insight into what the child is doing. In fact, he or she might be doing something that makes you anxious, and your defense is boredom or tiredness. In summary, your fleeting thoughts and subjective reactions are significant because they are part of the interactive matrix with a particular child at a given time.

SUMMARY

The categories I have been discussing in this chapter systematize and thereby stretch the potential implications of the observations you make when you meet a child in clinical interviews. As I explained at the start, multiple perspectives are necessary because behavior is so complicated and based on so many variables that the only way to get an understanding of it is to learn how to look at many dimensions simultaneously. Such an approach will keep you alert to the fact that any behavior can be based on a number of factors at once. I think it is an error to try to simplify prematurely by saying that a certain behavior belongs to only one category, such as the child's relatedness to the interviewer. In truth, this same behavior may be appropriately considered in several different frameworks.

Even a 3-minute capsule of a child's nonverbal behavior, observed from behind a one-way screen, for example, will yield a good initial picture of certain components of that child's personality and problems if you look at it from many different angles. What do the 3 minutes reveal about the child's physical and neurological integrity? Was the child coordinated? Does she show any gross motor incoordination? How is her fine motor coordination? What kind of activity did she engage in, and what was the activity level during those 3 minutes? Was the child hyperactive? Even if the child *was* hyperactive, you would want to observe more before making a hypothesis, for you do not know that the child always behaves that way.

You can also observe the emotional tone (e.g., the child seemed depressed, almost tearful), which is a clue to the child's overall mood. If, during the 3-minute interval, the child was clinging to the diagnostician, almost pleading for some kind of emotional contact and attention, that behavior may give you a sense of the degree of relatedness the child demands. You will also be able to observe the degree to which the child uses gestures in simple and complex ways, whether she is representational (using words or pretend) and/or representationally differentiated (using words and pretend in a logical manner). In such a time-limited situation you will not have the child's thematic development to augment your observations, but you may experience a clear-cut subjective reaction that should be taken into account. Thus, even in a 3-minute segment, with only a few specific pieces of behavior to observe, you are able to develop hypotheses based on multiple perspectives.

3

Chronological Age- and Phase- Appropriate Illustrations for Each Observational Category

IN THIS CHAPTER I will further illustrate the age- and phase-appropriate differences in the categories just described by means of a schematic chart. We will see that, for example, both the fine and the gross motor coordination of a 7- or 8-year-old are quite different from those of a 2- to 3-year-old. In a 2- or 3-year-old, coordination in gross motor capacities may already be developed, whereas some fine motor capacities will be just emerging (e.g., holding a pencil and drawing lines). By 7 or 8, in contrast, fine motor skills will be quite developed. With respect to style of relatedness, you would expect a 3-year-old to relate in a need-fulfilling manner, whereas you would expect a 7- or 8-year-old to show a more balanced capacity for partnership and sharing. In both instances, however, you would expect the capacity for emotional relatedness to be present.

In terms of mood, you might expect to see variations in the younger children depending on their immediate external circumstances. A shift from elation to sadness in the course of an hour would not raise concern. By 8 or 9 years old, in contrast, you would expect some stabilization of mood. At the same time, the content of the mood—happy, sad, depressed, apprehensive, and so forth—would be independent of age and would be determined by the emerging personality structure of the youngster.

In terms of the organization, depth, variation, and (predominant) types of affect, age will be a determining factor. With a 2- or 3-year-old, we might see affects concerned with egocentric needs, jealousies, and so forth. By age 5 or 6 we expect a range of affects, with predominant types reflecting some degree of organization and depth around themes of jealousy and competition, as well as love and curiosity. By 8 or 9 years of age we expect to see still further development in the affective system and perhaps an emerging capacity for experiencing empathy, sadness, tenderness, and compassion together with the affects from earlier stages.

We may also expect differences depending on age in the organization, richness, depth, and sequence of themes. In 3- and 4-year-olds, for example, thematic organization will be limited: the child may dramatically shift themes without logical links. By ages 5 and 6 we begin to see greater cohesion, although we are not surprised by "a theme seeming to jump out of left field." By 8 years of age, in contrast, we expect to see an organized elaboration of themes joined together by simple logical links.

In addition to observing how the child's capacities for organizing affects, emotional themes, and relationships meet age-appropriate expectations, it is important to emphasize that each of these categories of functioning is derived from the more general developmental levels described earlier. In Table 3-1, it can be seen how relationships can be organized in terms of the earliest and most basic aspects of engagement, can use two-way gestural communication (simple or complex), and/or can be characterized by the ability to symbolize or represent wishes, needs, and feelings as these emerge in the interactions at a particular age. Similarly, as a part of relationships, the communication of differentiated feelings and complex (gray-area) themes ("I'm sort of mad but also sort of like the person, too") can also be observed. Affects can also be seen to be expressed in terms of overall somatic states, in interactive gestures, in pretend play, in the functional use of language, and in differentiated representational forms, as illustrated by cause-and-effect thinking.

For each area of development—physical capacities, mood, relationships, affects, anxieties and fears, and thematic organization content and sequence—the general developmental model presented earlier will be the foundation for our understanding of how each area of functioning evolves. Table 3-1 therefore provides a road map for multiple aspects of development. This road map can be used to monitor normal, healthy development and to detect maladaptive or pathologic patterns.

This road map, it should be pointed out, differs from the more typical developmental tables that one sees in child development texts. The more typical tables present a road map for motor development, language, and/or certain selected social skills. In this road map, while we outline cognitive and social skills, we present aspects of development that are usually thought of as too ill-defined or vague for systematic explication. Furthermore, this road map presents those aspects of development that are the most relevant to the clinician: how a child relates, organizes his or her affects and mood, organizes his or her thinking, and so forth. Historically, these most clinically relevant dimensions of behavior, thought, and feeling have remained illusive. It is therefore hoped that this systematic presentation of clinically relevant aspects of development will prove valuable to clinicians in monitoring and understanding the clinical interview with the child.

Table 3-1 systematically illustrates age-appropriate differences in each category.

Table 3-1. A developmental approach to observing children: birth through age 10—1st year

Observational categories	1st year
1. *Physical functioning: neurological, sensory, motor integrative* Includes characteristic observations pertaining to the physical aspects of the child having to do with mental and psychological functioning, with special focus on the level of integration of the central nervous system, e.g., gross and fine motor coordination, perceptual-motor integration, emerging cognitive capacities.	Normal milestones, including turning toward stimulus, capacity to grab item in midline, sitting up, turning over, standing and eventually beginning to walk, clearer vocalizations, possibly a word or two (e.g., mama, dada), simple causal means-ends relationships with inanimate and animate world. Shows progress toward responding to social cues rather than internal sensations by 4 months. Increasing capacity to focus, comprehend, and concentrate as development progresses, associated with being interested (without hypo- or hyperactivity) in all age-appropriate sensations (e.g., touch, sound, sights, movement), and being able to process increasingly complex information in each sensory modality.
2. *Pattern of relationships* Includes characteristic style of relating or nonrelating (e.g., withdrawn, autistic), patterns of nonrelating, dyadic relating, capacity for group relating and sharing, egocentric styles of relating, etc.	General need for protection and comfort; multimodal interest in world evolves into highly individualized, pleasurable engagement and interactive (reciprocal) affective relationship with primary caregivers.
3. *Overall mood or emotional tone* Based on direct observation of specific emotions as well as themes or topics the child discusses. Characteristic patterns of this category may not be as clearly defined for each age group as those of the other categories.	Highly variable. Intimately related to internal states (e.g., hunger), and toward second half of first year also related to external social cues (parent can get even a hungry infant to smile). When internally comfortable, sense of interest and pleasure in world and in primary caregivers (e.g., drunken-sailor smile) should prevail.
4. *Affects* Consideration of: a. *Range and variety of affect:* the number of affects the child manifests: e.g., during early developmental phases range is limited or narrow; later the range is broader. Also includes characteristic types of affects: rage, jealousy, anger, empathy, love. b. *Depth of affect expression:* substantive nature of affects manifested: shallow versus substantive, etc. c. *Appropriateness of affect,* particularly in relationship to overall mood and content. d. *Discriminative capacity of affects:* to what degree can the affects be highly discriminative of specific feeling states? e. *Relationship of intensity of affect to stimulation or capacity for regulation of affect.*	Variation between indifference and excitement with world becomes more organized and under control of social interaction. Specific initial affects of pleasurable excitement and unpleasurable protest lead to more differentiated gradations of both pleasure and protest and apprehension (e.g., mild, moderate) and include gestures negotiating dependency, pleasure, assertiveness, exploration, anger, fear, and anxiety. Affect system remains highly variable and is easily dominated by context.

5. *Anxieties and fears*

Best observed either directly in child's verbalized fears or indirectly through play. Anxiety in particular can be observed by disruptions in thematic development either during play or conversation. Level of anxiety can be indicated by nature of the disruption and themes that follow it, e.g., anxieties around fear of physical injury; or of more global, undifferentiated types such as fear of loss, world destruction, or fragmentation of one's inner self.

Anxiety is usually global and disorganizing. Underlying concern hypothesized to be related to themes of annihilation, loss of emerging self and world.

6. *Thematic expression*

Includes the capacity to express organized, developmentally appropriate, rich themes. How well can the child communicate his or her personality to another, either indirectly through play or directly through verbal communication? Clearly, some children develop such a capacity in time because their basic sense of trust in the world, their security about their own inner controls, and the availability of their fantasy life enable them to communicate a rich feeling and content sense of themselves. Other children, by comparison, will be disorganized in their thematic expression (or very constricted, fragmented, impulsive, etc.). To subdivide thematic expression further, consider it from the following perspectives:

a. *Organization of thematic expression*: e.g., similar to organized or fragmented thinking.

b. *Depth and richness of thematic development.*

c. *Relevance in age-appropriate context*: How typical is content of themes to age-appropriate concerns?

d. *Thematic sequence.* This can be used in describing children at each age.

Behavior related to internal cues evolves into simple social, purposeful causal behavioral chains (e.g., mother smiles, baby reaches out with hand to elicit a similar response from mother) and simple reciprocal or contingent behavior. Capacity for organized, reciprocal interactions (e.g., mother smiles and baby smiles) to more complex chains of interaction toward end of first year (e.g., reaching out, holding object, and giving it to mother). Social interactions involve themes of pleasure, exploration, and protest.

Table 3-1—2nd year

Observational categories	2nd year
1. Physical functioning: neurological, sensory, motor integrative Includes characteristic observations pertaining to the physical aspects of the child having to do with mental and psychological functioning, with special focus on the level of integration of the central nervous system, e.g., gross and fine motor coordination, perceptual-motor integration, emerging cognitive capacities.	Normal milestones, including clumsy to coordinated walking and even running, climbing steps, etc. Fine motor capacities increasing (e.g., can scribble). Increasing comprehension of complex gestures and simple words and phrases. Growing ability to communicate with gestures and words across space. Vocalizations becoming more distinct with capacity to name many objects and make needs known in two words: and near end of second year into third year, using sentences. Capacity for developing new behaviors from old ones (originality) and emerging capacity for symbolic activity (e.g., using words to describe self and others, play with dolls); variable capacity for concentration and self-regulation.
2. Pattern of relationships Includes characteristic style of relating or nonrelating (e.g., withdrawn, autistic), patterns of nonrelating, dyadic relating, capacity for group relating and sharing, egocentric styles of relating, etc.	Dyadic relationship with primary caregivers evolves into a balance between need fulfillment (basic dependency) and emerging individuality, autonomy, initiative, and capacity for self-organization at the behavioral level (e.g., the toddler who goes to the refrigerator to get what he or she wants). Some negativism may be present. Issues of need and concerns with separation still paramount.
3. Overall mood or emotional tone Based on direct observation of specific emotions as well as themes or topics the child discusses. Characteristic patterns of this category may not be as clearly defined for each age group as those of the other categories.	Also variable, but more organized and stable for longer periods of time. Sense of security, curiosity, and exploration should dominate over moods of emotional hunger, the tendency to cling, negativism, fear, and/or apprehension. A basic mood may be beginning to emerge.
4. Affects Consideration of: a. *Range and variety of affect:* the number of affects the child manifests: e.g., during early developmental phases range is limited or narrow; later the range is broader. Also includes characteristic types of affects: rage, jealousy, anger, empathy, love. b. *Depth of affect expression:* substantive nature of affects manifested: shallow versus substantive, etc. c. *Appropriateness of affect,* particularly in relationship to overall mood and content. d. *Discriminative capacity of affects:* to what degree can the affects be highly discriminative of specific feeling states? e. *Relationship of intensity of affect to stimulation or capacity for regulation of affect.*	Affects become further differentiated. Observed are excited explorations, assertive pleasure, pleasure in discovery. More complex gestural negotiations of dependency, assertiveness, anger, and self-limit-setting. Capacity for organized demonstration of love (e.g., running up and hugging, smiling, and kissing parent—all together) and protest (e.g., turning away, crying, banging, and kicking—all together). Organized negativism (the no's) and clinging demandingness also present. Balance should be in direction of organized expressions of pleasure in discovery, initiative, and love. Comfort with family and apprehension with strangers may be more developed.

5. Anxieties and fears

Best observed either directly in child's verbalized fears or indirectly through play. Anxiety in particular can be observed by disruptions in thematic development either during play or conversation. Level of anxiety can be indicated by nature of the disruption and themes that follow it, e.g., anxieties around fear of physical injury; or of more global, undifferentiated types such as fear of loss, world destruction, or fragmentation of one's inner self.

Anxiety related to loss of loved caretaker—potentially disorganizing.

6. Thematic expression

Includes the capacity to express organized, developmentally appropriate, rich themes. How well can child communicate his or her personality to another, either indirectly through play or directly through verbal communication? Clearly, some children develop such a capacity in time because their basic sense of trust in the world, their security about their own inner controls, and the availability of their fantasy life enable them to communicate a rich feeling and content sense of themselves. Other children, by comparison, will be disorganized in their thematic expression (or very constricted, fragmented, impulsive, etc.). To subdivide thematic expression further, consider it from the following perspectives:

a. *Organization of thematic expression:* e.g., similar to organized or fragmented thinking.

b. *Depth and richness of thematic development.*

c. *Revelance in age-appropriate context.* How typical is content of themes to age-appropriate concerns?

d. *Thematic sequence.* This can be used in describing children at each age.

Capacity for organization of behavior into complex causal chains (e.g., taking mother by hand to refrigerator and showing her desired food); initiative and originality at behavioral level as well as increased initiative behavior. At behavioral level child reflects themes of love, curiosity, exploration and protest, anger, negativism, and jealousy—all in organized modes (e.g., running to father and hugging and kissing him as one organized series; or turning away, throwing down toy, and screaming as another). Toward end of second year emerging capacities to *integrate* themes that reflect *polarities* of love and anger, passivity and activity, emerging, e.g., in one game—"The doll is bad, gets spanked, and then is hugged." Also emerging representational or symbolic capacities in relationships and emotional themes.

67

Table 3-1—3rd year

Observational categories	3rd year
1. Physical functioning: neurological, sensory, motor integrative Includes characteristic observations pertaining to the physical aspects of the child having to do with mental and psychological functioning, with special focus on the level of integration of the central nervous system, e.g., gross and fine motor coordination, perceptual-motor integration, emerging cognitive capacities.	Coordinated gross motor activity: running, walking up and down stairs without holding on, etc. Fine motor coordination more differentiated (e.g., can scribble circles, hold feeding utensils). Can comprehend phrases and simple sentences and complex gestures. Can name many objects, use personal pronouns and sentences to describe events, and make needs known. Symbolic capacity expanded as evidenced in wider fantasy life (e.g., dreams, fears, make-believe stories and people); capacity for concentration and self-regulation still variable but improving.
2. Pattern of relationships Includes characteristic style of relating or nonrelating (e.g., withdrawn, autistic), patterns of nonrelating, dyadic relating, capacity for group relating and sharing, egocentric styles of relating, etc.	Relationships, though still dyadic and need-fulfilling, now become organized at a representational or symbolic level (i.e., a sense of self and other in terms of thoughts, memories, etc., is emerging) and permit use of fantasy. Balance between dependency and autonomy may shift for a brief time to the former. Power struggles and negativism may intermittently dominate relationship pattern. Dominant issues continue to be basic dependency and the need for security, and fear of separation. Symbolic interactions in power, control, aggression, and different types of pleasure in relationships emerging. Capacity for more complex interactions since internal imagery can now be used (e.g., language or a doll used to represent needs in a complex game).
3. Overall mood or emotional tone Based on direct observation of specific emotions as well as themes or topics the child discusses. Characteristic patterns of this category may not be as clearly defined for each age group as those of the other categories.	Initially may become quite variable (e.g., moody, fussy, and clinging behavior together with secure explorativeness), but then gradually stabilizes into even pattern organized around a basic sense of security and optimism, with capacity for excitement, negativism, passivity, tendency to cling, etc., present but not dominant.
4. Affects Consideration of: a. *Range and variety of affect*: the number of affects the child manifests: e.g., during early developmental phases range is limited or narrow; later the range is broader. Also includes characteristic types of affects: rage, jealousy, anger, empathy, love. b. *Depth of affect expression*: substantive nature of affects manifested: shallow versus substantive, etc. c. *Appropriateness of affect*, particularly in relationship to overall mood and content.	Affects now gradually have more "meaning" (representational or symbolic level). After possible initial instability in affect system (e.g., regressive, clinging anger and dependency), greater organization of affect system possible, with such complex affects as love, unhappiness, jealousy, and envy expressed at both preverbal and emerging verbal level. Affect system still easily influenced by somatic events (e.g., tiredness, hunger). Affects still mostly at egocentric level ("What's in it for me").

d. *Discriminative capacity of affects*: to what degree can the affects be highly discriminative of specific feeling states?

e. *Relationship of intensity of affect to stimulation or capacity for regulation of affect.*

5. *Anxieties and fears*

Best observed either directly in child's verbalized fears or indirectly through play. Anxiety in particular can be observed by disruptions in thematic development either during play or conversation. Level of anxiety can be indicated by nature of the disruption and themes that follow it, e.g., anxieties around fear of physical injury; or of more global, undifferentiated types such as fear of loss, world destruction, or fragmentation of one's inner self.

6. *Thematic expression*

Includes the capacity to express organized, developmentally appropriate, rich themes. How well can child communicate his or her personality to another, either indirectly through play or directly through verbal communication? Clearly, some children develop such a capacity in time because their basic sense of trust in the world, their security about their own inner controls, and the availability of their fantasy life enable them to communicate a rich feeling and content sense of themselves. Other children, by comparison, will be disorganized in their thematic expression (or very constricted, fragmented, impulsive, etc.). To subdivide thematic expression further, consider it from the following perspectives:

a. *Organization of thematic expression*: e.g., similar to organized or fragmented thinking.

b. *Depth and richness of thematic development.*

c. *Relevance in age-appropriate context*: How typical is content of themes to age-appropriate concerns?

d. *Thematic sequence.* This can be used in describing children at each age.

Anxiety related to loss of loved and depended-on person as well as loss of approval and acceptance. While still potentially disorganizing, anxiety can be better tolerated and may be coped with through alterations in mental imagery (fantasy) (e.g., "Mother will be back, she loves me").

Behavior remains organized as in second year, and even more complex chains of interaction are possible. Now symbolic or representational capacity, as evidenced by language and use of personal pronouns (I, you, etc.), and elaboration of fantasy through language and behavior (e.g., play in which child has one doll, mother another doll) emerge. In contrast to *organized* behavior, symbolic communication is initially fragmented (e.g., seemingly disconnected islands of pretend play or verbal communication). There is a gradual elaboration of experience—simple repetitive themes, "Want that," or pretend play of dolls hugging leads to a broad range of themes concerning power, pleasure, dependency, fear, etc. These themes gradually become more complex (e.g., the dolls hug and then kiss). Themes involve repeating what is seen and heard, exploring inanimate and animate world with new symbolic capacities, and then using symbolic modes for emotional interaction. There is a vacillation between attempts at self-definition—through trying to be in "control," power struggles, negativism, and joyful and excited development of new behavior and thoughts (discovery at the symbolic level)—and regressive dependent interests (holding, clinging, etc.), which, however, also have the element of "I'm in control." Improving capacity for self-control and responding to limits and structure at symbolic level. Interest in theme of power (e.g., rocket ships, powerful heros, pretending to be a monster and being scared of monsters) emerges toward end of third year.

Table 3-1—4th year

Observational categories	4th year
1. *Physical functioning: neurological, sensory, motor integrative* Includes characteristic observations pertaining to the physical aspects of the child having to do with mental and psychological functioning, with special focus on the level of integration of the central nervous system, e.g., gross and fine motor coordination, perceptual-motor integration, emerging cognitive capacities.	Gross motor coordination continues to improve; child can run, jump, hop, throw a ball accurately, etc. Fine motor coordination improves, e.g., child can almost tie shoes, can draw circles, handles utensils very well. Comprehends two or more connected concepts or ideas. Can talk in full sentences, connecting ideas with words like "but" and "because," and make needs known. Symbolic capacity not only expanded (e.g., complex play with dolls) but ability for reality orientation (distinguishing fantasy from reality) increasing; concentration and self-regulation possible with appropriate context and support.
2. *Pattern of relationships* Includes characteristic style of relating or nonrelating (e.g., withdrawn, autistic), patterns of nonrelating, dyadic relating, capacity for group relating and sharing, egocentric styles of relating, etc.	Relationship patterns becoming more complicated not only in content (language, symbolic modes) but in form, as dyadic patterns begin to recede and capacities for dealing with triangular and other more complicated patterns emerge (e.g., rivalries, intrigues, secrets, two against one, jealousies, envy). Capacity for peer relationships increasing as well. Greater sense of security; capacity for separation and for carrying sense of the "other" inside relatively well established by end of fourth year. Anger and other strong feelings do not compromise secure capacity for separation. Capacity for intimacy (not simply need-fulfilling) in relationships emerging more fully.
3. *Overall mood or emotional tone* Based on direct observation of specific emotions as well as themes or topics the child discusses. Characteristic patterns of this category may not be as clearly defined for each age group as those of the other categories.	Mood stabilizes further and organizes complex feelings; less extreme reactions to frustration (e.g., having to delay). Basic attitude toward self and world conveyed in organized mood, which optimally reflects security in psychological and bodily self and curious expansive interest with excitement in family, peers, and the world. Insecurity and negativism receding in importance.
4. *Affects* Consideration of: a. *Range and variety of affect:* the number of affects the child manifests: e.g., during early developmental phases range is limited or narrow; later the range is broader. Also includes characteristic types of affects: rage, jealousy, anger, empathy, love. b. *Depth of affect expression:* Substantive nature of affects manifested: shallow versus substantive, etc. c. *Appropriateness of affect,* particularly in relationship to overall mood and content.	Pride and joy in psychological and bodily self further emerge. Increased interest in power; affects of shame and humiliation become dominant. Increased feelings of jealousy and envy; more differentiated sadistic and masochistic trends. Emerging capacity for sharing and concern for others. Empathy and tenderness increasing. Affect system well organized, showing large number of affect states of the emerging sense of self.

d. *Discriminative capacity of affects:* to what degree can the affects be highly discriminative of specific feeling states?

e. *Relationship of intensity of affect to stimulation or capacity for regulation of affect.*

5. Anxieties and fears

Best observed either directly in child's verbalized fears or indirectly through play. Anxiety in particular can be observed by disruptions in thematic development either during play or conversation. Level of anxiety can be indicated by nature of the disruption and themes that follow it, e.g., anxieties around fear of physical injury; or of more global, undifferentiated types such as fear of loss, world destruction, or fragmentation of one's inner self.

Anxiety over loss of loved person's approval and bodily injury sometimes disruptive, but usually not. Multiple fears of being robbed, kidnapped, hurt, or parents being taken away or hurt not uncommon, but usually understood as either "only a dream" or "not real."

6. Thematic expression

Includes the capacity to express organized, developmentally appropriate, rich themes. How well can child communicate his or her personality to another, either indirectly through play or directly through verbal communication? Clearly, some children develop such a capacity in time because their basic sense of trust in the world, their security about their own inner controls, and the availability of their fantasy life enable them to communicate a rich feeling and content sense of themselves. Other children, by comparison, will be disorganized in their thematic expression (or very constricted, fragmented, impulsive, etc.). To subdivide thematic expression further, consider it from the following perspectives:

a. *Organization of thematic expression:* e.g., similar to organized or fragmented thinking.

b. *Depth and richness of thematic development.*

c. *Relevance in age-appropriate context.* How typical is content of themes to age-appropriate concerns?

d. *Thematic sequence.* This can be used in describing children at each age.

Thematic organization at behavioral level continues in a richer, more complex fashion. Now, however, complex themes at a symbolic level are also becoming organized compared to fragmentation of third year (e.g., organized verbal elaboration of fantasy now possible in the reporting of a dream: "A monster came in and was going to attack me, but then I punched him in the nose . . ." and in symbolic play: building a fort to protect dolls from the various monsters; having a "tea party," cooking various foods and serving guests). Some vacillation between these organized themes and fragmented ones, but indications of rich, organized inner life present. Content of themes a product of inner fantasy life. Capacity for reality orientation present as well—"that's just make-believe." Tendency is to be swept away by fantasy for short periods of time. In *circumscribed areas* fantasy may dominate reality over long periods, for example, in fears around going to sleep. Themes around both aggression- and pleasure-derived power and interest in and fear of the body dominate, together with curiosity, a sense of discovery, feelings of pride, admiration of self and others, and concerns with shame. Also present are concerns with security, fears of loss of love and separation, and power struggles and issues of control.

Table 3-1—5th and 6th years

Observational categories	5th and 6th years
1. *Physical functioning: neurological, sensory, motor integrative* Includes characteristic observations pertaining to the physical aspects of the child having to do with mental and psychological functioning, with special focus on the level of integration of the central nervous system, e.g., gross and fine motor coordination, perceptual-motor integration, emerging cognitive capacities.	Gross motor coordination improves, as evidenced by more accurate throwing, rhythmic jumping (rope), kicking (e.g., football). Fine motor coordination improves, e.g., ties shoes; writes letters; draws circles, squares, and triangles; talks in full, complex sentences; begins to demonstrate capacity to present ideas. Can begin to comprehend, express, and conceptualize simple reciprocal and inverse relationships between multiple ideas and aspects of physical reality (e.g., line up shapes according to length or figure out degrees of intensity of anger or greed). Capacity for self-regulation and concentration improving, but still subject to context and support.
2. *Pattern of relationships* Includes characteristic style of relating or nonrelating (e.g., withdrawn, autistic), patterns of nonrelating, dyadic relating, capacity for group relating and sharing, egocentric styles of relating, etc.	Complex triangular modes dominate family life as relationships take on "soap opera" dimensions of intrigue, rivalry, alliances, etc. Simple need-fulfilling two-person relationships pattern less dominant. Capacity to relate comfortably with others—peers, teachers—growing. Growing capacity for separation, internal security; ability to carry a sense of "self" and "other" inside not only well established but not easily compromised by separations or strong affects.
3. *Overall mood or emotional tone* Based on direct observation of specific emotions as well as themes or topics the child discusses. Characteristic patterns of this category may not be as clearly defined for each age group as those of the other categories.	Stable, organized mood characterized by expressiveness and curiosity. Variations in affect (e.g., fearfulness, inhibition, unwillingness to compromise), but overall organization and stability of mood.
4. *Affects* Consideration of: a. *Range and variety of affect:* the number of affects the child manifests: e.g., during early developmental phases range is limited or narrow; later the range is broader. Also includes characteristic types of affects: rage, jealousy, anger, empathy, love. b. *Depth of affect expression:* substantive nature of affects manifested: shallow versus substantive, etc. c. *Appropriateness of affect*, particularly in relationship to overall mood and content. d. *Discriminative capacity of affects:* to what degree can the affects be highly discriminative of specific feeling states? e. *Relationship of intensity of affect to stimulation or capacity for regulation of affect.*	Many individual affects in relatively stable pattern: expansiveness, curiousity, pride, gleeful excitement related to discovery of bodily self and family patterns; balanced with coyness, shyness, fearfulness, jealousy, and envy. Shame and humiliation still dominant. Capacity for empathy and love developed, but fragile and easily lost if competitive or jealous strivings are on the upsurge.

5. Anxieties and fears

Best observed directly in child's verbalized fears or indirectly through play. Anxiety in particular can be observed by disruptions in thematic development either during play or conversation. Level of anxiety can be indicated by nature of the disruption and themes that follow it, e.g., anxieties around fear of physical injury; or of more global, undifferentiated types such as fear of loss, world destruction, or fragmentation of one's inner self.

Anxiety and fears related to bodily injury and loss of respect, love, and emerging self-esteem; self-esteem may vacillate between extremes. Guilt feelings emerging.

6. Thematic expression

Includes the capacity to express organized, developmentally appropriate, rich themes. How well can child communicate his or her personality to another, either indirectly through play or directly through verbal communication? Clearly, some children develop such a capacity in time because their basic sense of trust in the world, their security about their own inner controls, and the availability of their fantasy life enable them to communicate a rich feeling and content sense of themselves. Other children, by comparison, will be disorganized in their thematic expression (or very constricted, fragmented, impulsive, etc.). To subdivide thematic expression further, consider it from the following perspectives:

a. *Organization of thematic expression*: e.g., similar to organized or fragmented thinking.

b. *Depth and richness of thematic development.*

c. *Relevance in age-appropriate context.* How typical is content of themes to age-appropriate concerns?

d. *Thematic sequence.* This can be used in describing children at each age.

Rich, organized, complex, symbolic thematic capacity with occasional fragmentation. While capable of being swept away by the fantasy, reality orientation well established. "That's not real" except at times in certain circumscribed areas around fears, etc. Content of themes represents rich, complex interest in major issues of the world: sex, aggression, power, curiosity, discovery, emerging morality, etc. Polarities of love, pleasure, and aggression should be present and integrated into complex, rich themes (e.g., game where child first takes care of sibling in a loving fashion, later becomes an attacking monster, and then becomes concerned with retaliation). For the first time, triangular patterns in relationships emerge in thematic expression—feeling left out, wishing to leave someone else out, game or fantasy of getting rid of "other" person in triangle, etc. Slight shift from interests in power and one's own body and how it compares to others', to real curiosity about others and their bodies and what goes on "behind closed doors." Fear of bodily injury takes over, although earlier fears of loss of approval and separation are present. Emerging fears of loss of own self-esteem now possible (e.g., "I am bad" or "I'm not good at anything").

73

Table 3-1—7th and 8th years

Observational categories	7th and 8th years
1. *Physical functioning; neurological, sensory, motor integrative* Includes characteristic observations pertaining to the physical aspects of the child having to do with mental and psychological functioning, with special focus on the level of integration of the central nervous system, e.g., gross and fine motor coordination, perceptual-motor integration, emerging cognitive capacities.	Gross motor coordination improves even further as child can now do most activities: running, jumping, hopping, skipping, throwing, etc. Fine motor coordination improves, as evidenced by being able to write more fluently in script, improved drawing, etc. Language used more and more in comprehending and communicating many interrelated ideas and concepts. Language used to present wishes, needs, and fantasies, as well as logical ideas oriented toward making orderly sense of the world. Capacity for logic in terms of inverse and reciprocal relationships established. Capacity for self-regulation, following rules, and concentrating established.
2. *Pattern of relationships* Includes characteristic style of relating or nonrelating (e.g., withdrawn, autistic), patterns of nonrelating, dyadic relating, capacity for group relating and sharing, egocentric styles of relating, etc.	Interest in relationships outside family groups (e.g., peers) and capacity for organized orderly patterns of relating to others (e.g., games with rules) emerge. Some aspects of earlier patterns still present, however (e.g., power struggles, passive helplessness, family intrigues, rivalries, triangles). Capacity for "buddy" and intimacy with a few "best" friends emerging more fully.
3. *Overall mood or emotional tone* Based on direct observation of specific emotions as well as themes or topics the child discusses. Characteristic patterns of this category may not be as clearly defined for each age group as those of the other categories.	Stable, organized mood characterized by emerging appraisal of self, others, and world, often based on perceptions of peer group, family group, and adults such as teachers and coaches. Expansive curiosity balanced with more sober, orderly approach.
4. *Affects* Consideration of: a. *Range and variety of affect*: the number of affects the child manifests: e.g., during early developmental phases range is limited or narrow; later the range is broader. Also includes characteristic types of affects: rage, jealousy, anger, empathy, love. b. *Depth of affect expression*: substantive nature of affects manifested: shallow versus substantive, etc. c. *Appropriateness of affect*, particularly in relationship to overall mood and content. d. *Discriminative capacity of affects*: to what degree can the affects be highly discriminative of specific feeling states? e. *Relationship of intensity of affect to stimulation or capacity for regulation of affect.*	Pleasure in approval, over success, and over mastery (self-esteem) emerge and operate in balance with the expansive and competitive affects described above and fear of failure and humiliation. Less variation in specific affects, though large number of affects still possible. Some instability between attempts to keep self in order and on right track (e.g., affects of self-praise, self-esteem) and earlier expansive and rivalrous affects. At times, earlier affects of envy, negativism, and egocentric emotional hunger pervade. Concern for others, empathy, and even worry growing.

5. Anxieties and fears

Best observed either directly in child's verbalized fears or indirectly through play. Anxiety in particular can be observed by disruptions in thematic development either during play or conversation. Level of anxiety can be indicated by nature of the disruption and themes that follow it, e.g., anxieties around fear of physical injury, or of more global, undifferentiated types such as fear of loss, world destruction, or fragmentation of one's inner self.

6. Thematic expression

Includes the capacity to express organized, developmentally appropriate, rich themes. How well can child communicate his or her personality to another, either indirectly through play or directly through verbal communication? Clearly, some children develop such a capacity in time because their basic sense of trust in the world, their security about their own inner controls, and the availability of their fantasy life enable them to communicate a rich feeling and content sense of themselves. Other children, by comparison, will be disorganized in their thematic expression (or very constricted, fragmented, impulsive, etc.). To subdivide thematic expression further, consider it from the following perspectives:

a. *Organization of thematic expression:* e.g., similar to organized or fragmented thinking.

b. *Depth and richness of thematic development.*

c. *Relevance in age-appropriate context.* How typical is content of themes to age-appropriate concerns?

d. *Thematic sequence.* This can be used in describing children at each age.

Anxiety is occasionally disruptive, usually serves a signal function and can be dealt with via shift in fantasy or change in meanings (e.g., reaction formations). Fears of humiliation or shame, loss of respect, and disapproval dominate (e.g., "They think I am terrible at soccer," "Everyone hates me"), with earlier fears of loss of love, separation, and bodily injury still present. Guilt feelings present ("I am bad"), but often dependent on context.

Relatively rich, organized thematic development with perhaps slightly less richness or breadth than in 5- to 6-year-old period, but more organized with less fragmentation. Less emphasis now on expanding interest in world, triangles, intrigues, the human body, what goes on behind closed doors, and various aggressive themes (monsters, attacking, etc.); more emphasis on containing these interests (e.g., "I'm not interested in what's going on behind the door, let me look and I'll show you I'm not interested"). In sense of polarities, there is a slight shift from pleasurable pursuits toward themes of control but balance should still be present. Interest in "roles" (what I am—"a football player," etc.) emerging as more dominant. Activity and assertion should be better modulated (e.g., regulates self and follows instructions). Occasional passive compliance may be present. Sense of morality (what's right and wrong) emerging but still unstable. Concern with rules and structure emerging; relatively greater interest in peers and the group, and slightly diminished interest in the family and adults.

Greenspan, S. I. (1991). The clinical interview of the child (2nd ed.). Washington, DC: American Psychiatric Press, Inc.

Table 3-1—9th and 10th years

Observational categories	9th and 10th years
1. Physical functioning: *neurological, sensory, motor integrative* Includes characteristic observations pertaining to the physical aspects of the child having to do with mental and psychological functioning, with special focus on the level of integration of the central-nervous system, e.g., gross and fine motor coordination, perceptual-motor integration, emerging cognitive capacities.	Greater muscle strength enhances gross motor coordination: gradual further improvement in all areas, with the capacity for complex activities (e.g., basketball, football, tennis). New learning more established. Fine motor coordination also improves, with more fluid writing and the capacity to take things apart (e.g., with screwdriver) skillfully. Language now used to comprehend and express complex ideas with relationships among a number of elements, e.g., "I did this because he did that, and he did that because she made him." Able to use logic to understand gradations in feelings or aspects of physical reality and more complex inverse and reciprocal relationships. Tendency for logical exploration to dominate fantasy; greater sense of morality; increased interest in rules and orderliness; increased capacity for self-regulation; well established ability to concentrate.
2. Pattern of relationships Includes characteristic style of relating or nonrelating (e.g., withdrawn, autistic), patterns of nonrelating, dyadic relating, capacity for group relating and sharing, egocentric styles of relating, etc. *Social - cog. dev.*	Peer relationships continue to grow in importance and complexity. Family relationships and friendships may be organized around role models (e.g., simplified adult stereotypes). Relaxed capacity for integrating and enjoying family, peer, teacher, and other adult relationships. Special relationship with same-sex parent as role model, with only hints of earlier levels (e.g., triangles, power struggles, passive manipulation). Preparation for adolescent styles of relating emerging, with special patterns of relating to same- and opposite-sex peers. Capacity for *long-term* relationships with family, peers, and friends—including "best friend(s)." Less reactive to day-to-day peer fluctuations toward end of 10th year.
3. Overall mood or emotional tone Based on direct observation of specific emotions as well as themes or topics the child discusses. Characteristic patterns of this category may not be as clearly defined for each age group as those of the other categories.	Stability, depth, and organization of mood further developed, as evidenced by capacity to deal with frustration, complex interpersonal relationships, etc., with sense of curiosity and *realistic* optimism (which is gradually replacing expansiveness). Overwhelming sadness, negativism, passive helplessness, and withdrawn moods should only emerge intermittently (e.g., in appropriate circumstances of stress).
4. Affects Consideration of: a. *Range and variety of affect:* the number of affects the child manifests: e.g., during early developmental phases range is limited or narrow; later the range is broader. Also includes characteristic types of affects: rage, jealousy, anger, empathy, love.	Well-developed capacity for empathy, love, compassion, sharing, and emerging capacity for sadness and loss in context of concrete rules. Internal self-esteem very important. Feelings of guilt and internalized fears present. Expansive lust, hunger, and jealousy in background. New affects around sexual differences beginning to emerge (e.g., excitement and shyness in relation to sexual themes).

76

b. *Depth of affect expression:* substantive nature of affects manifested: shallow versus substantive, etc.

c. *Appropriateness of affect,* particularly in relationship to overall mood and content.

d. *Discriminative capacity of affects:* to what degree can the affects be highly discriminative of specific feeling states?

e. *Relationship of intensity of affect to stimulation or capacity for regulation of affect.*

5. *Anxieties and fears*

Best observed either directly in child's verbalized fears or indirectly through play. Anxiety in particular can be observed by disruptions in thematic development either during play or conversation. Level of anxiety can be indicated by nature of the disruption and themes that follow it, e.g., anxieties around fear of physical injury; or of more global, undifferentiated types such as fear of loss, world destruction, or fragmentation of one's inner self.

Anxiety related to internalized conflicts generally not disruptive; may be dysphoric and/or serve a signal function and lead to change in behavior, interpretation of events, or more sophisticated changes in meanings and fantasies (e.g., rationalizations). Fears of loss of self-esteem related to loss of respect, humiliation, and shame are still present. Fear of one's own guilt growing stronger ("I can't do that. It will make me feel bad").

6. *Thematic expression*

Includes the capacity to express organized, developmentally appropriate, rich themes. How well can child communicate his or her personality to another, either indirectly through play or directly through verbal communication? Clearly, some children develop such a capacity in time because their basic sense of trust in the world, their security about their own inner controls, and the availability of their fantasy life enable them to communicate a rich feeling and content sense of themselves. Other children, by comparison, will be disorganized in their thematic expression (or very constricted, fragmented, impulsive, etc.). To subdivide thematic expression further, consider it from the following perspectives:

a. *Organization of thematic expression:* e.g., similar to organized or fragmented thinking.

b. *Depth and richness of thematic development.*

c. *Relevance in age-appropriate context.* How typical is content of themes to age-appropriate concerns?

d. *Thematic sequence.* This can be used in describing children at each age.

Thematic capacity quite well organized, e.g., capable of relating organized story about the robbers who are caught by the policemen in great detail, with elaborations of the robbers' plans and how the policemen fooled them. Stories of football games or parties where adult roles are imitated are also presented in a detailed, organized manner. Little or no fragmentation as more and more interrelated detail can be organized. Some of the emotional richness and complexity of the 5- or 6-year-old phase relinquished for greater interest in themes around control, rules, organization, and higher-level domination-submission themes. The new interest in "roles" and "what I will be" and "how good I am at this or that" or "how bad I am at this or that," and differences between boys and girls emerging. Variable interest in talking both with peers and, somewhat sheepishly, with adults about sex (e.g., dirty jokes with giggling) in anticipation of adolescence. Concerns with self-regard and how others regard one are also prominent. Internal morality relatively well established in concrete "black and white" sense, but still easy to rationalize breaking the rules. In fact, along with greater concern with right and wrong is more sophisticated capacity for rationalizing and getting around the rules. Self-control and capacity to follow instructions should be quite well established, however.

4

Clinical Illustrations of Interviews With Children

THE CLINICAL DESCRIPTIONS presented below—interview patterns developed by 18 young children—were constructed from brief process notes that I made after each interview. The reader may wish to read these illustrative examples and then attempt to organize the data according to the categories outlined earlier. A first-level clinical inference may then be attempted in terms of describing whether each category of functioning is at the appropriate age level or below it. In Chapter 6 I will discuss the elaboration of these inferences into clinical hypotheses. It should be emphasized that the single clinical interview, while a vital component, is only one part of an evaluation process. Other components include additional interviews, developmental history, descriptions of current functioning, family patterns, school reports and observations, and medical, neurological, psychological, sensory, motor, cognitive, and language studies as needed. In this book the focus is only on the clinical interview.

CASE 1

Interview

Doug was a well-groomed, average-sized boy of 8½ years. He was sitting on a chair next to his mother in the waiting room, doodling on a pad that he had brought with him. He looked up with a blank expression when I asked him to join me, and readily came into the office with me. He had a somewhat sober, perhaps even sad look about him. He made ready eye contact, however, was well coordinated, and walked in an easygoing fashion. He sat on the couch and, without saying a word, scribbled on his pad. His fine motor coordination looked good; he was able to manipulate the pen well. He was right-handed.

During a brief, mildly uncomfortable pause, as I waited to see if he would begin communication, it appeared that he was almost frozen with silence. He just sat there. After I saw that he was not about to break the silence, I commented that he liked to draw and doodle. He quickly responded that it was okay to doodle, but he had no strong feelings about it one way or another. I then sat down next to him and noticed that he was drawing a cartoon figure. The profiled face had a square nose and a big mouth, with the word "Hi" coming out of it. The figure had a trunk but no legs. I commented that Doug seemed to like to draw cartoons; he quickly replied that it was his brother who really liked to draw cartoons.

Doug pointed out that he ran errands, going to the store for groceries and the like, and then elaborated about how he had started a little business. His family lived in an apartment and for a quarter he would do errands for other families in the building. At this point in the interview he started getting affectively excited and emotionally involved. "They give me big tips," he said. "I got a dollar today for going shopping for a lady." He then related with pleasure and pride that he had made $30 in the last month, and that when he made $30 more, he would have $560 in the bank and then he would have "enough" money.

I was curious about what the money was for and what he meant by "enough" money. He said, "Enough is for the future, in case of an emergency." I said, "There are a lot of different kinds of emergencies." (It is best not to ask questions of children—e.g., "What kind of an emergency are you worried about?" It is more constructive simply to comment empathically about their concerns.) In response to my remark, Doug said only that it is always good to have money because there are all kinds of emergencies. He did not develop the theme more specifically, but did make side comments about inflation, world conditions, and the selling of airplanes to Arabs.

As he talked to me, Doug became more relaxed and looked more often in my direction. Although his voice reflected a degree of sadness and a narrow affective range, he showed generally increasing interest, some pleasure, and particularly some pride as he talked about his business interest and making money for the future. His verbal communication was well organized; that is, he chose a topic and discussed it without getting lost or going off on a tangent. He illustrated his topic—how important it was to be a good businessman—with pertinent examples.

The money theme, in various modes, permeated the interview. It was not good, he told me, to "buy lots of toys now, because it is better to have money for later." He told me about schoolmates who spent all their money on toys and said that he did not do that. Upon inquiry he told me that he learned this from his parents, that his whole family was very concerned with "saving money." (The boy's father is an extraordinarily successful author.)

He then told me about "lazy bums who live in the street and don't work, and don't have money or a place to sleep." I commented that this sounded kind of sad and unfortunate. He replied that he was not sympathetic, that they were lazy and it was their problem that they could not earn money. He seemed annoyed at their laziness. He also said that these people may be "stupid" as well as lazy, and that they do not take care of themselves. He went on with the theme of people who do not take care of themselves or plan for the future. Whenever I commented that he seemed to be just the opposite, he appeared very pleased and further elaborated about these lazy people. He told me spontaneously what he was worried would happen: something to do with an emergency and with why he was not like these lazy people. I was curious what he thought these lazy people who lie in the street were like. I began, "Gee, there are all kinds of lazy people who don't take care of themselves," and continued free-associating for half a minute about "lazy bums." Then he told me, "Well, a lot of them are 'robbers,' these 'lazy bums.' "

During this time he made relatively good eye contact and affective engagement. He was unusual in that he talked a blue streak and did not explore the room, staying focused on the issues of protecting oneself from future emergencies and lazy bums.

Next he talked about robbers coming into the house and how his little brother (who is 2½ years old) would not know what to do and would get hurt. He then abruptly returned to the topic of future emergencies and began to clarify what he meant by emergencies. He spoke of people getting sick, having cancer and other illnesses that people die from, and said that you never know when you are going to die. Then he talked briefly about his older brother and what his older brother is better at than he is, and about his younger brother, saying that the latter was a pest. However, he added that he was learning to adjust to the younger brother and did not really want to get rid of him. He returned to the subject of physical illness and became preoccupied with it. He associated in a free-wheeling and unusually open manner, almost like someone lying on the couch. There was no sense of his being guarded about what he was saying. His affect during these disclosures was reasonably engaging with a mildly hungry quality.

Near the end of the session he expressed a worry from out of the blue. He asked if his older brother would know what we were talking about; that is, if the session was tape-recorded, could his brother find out? He quickly changed his mind about this, saying, "No, that's silly, that's not possible"; then he wondered if we could do things together, play basketball or tennis.

When I asked about his family, he became very anxious. He mentioned something about the things he liked to do with his father, such as play ball. (I knew that his father had a serious heart disease.) When discussing his activities with father, Doug got to the issue of his father's physical limitations and became acutely anxious, freezing for a second and then changing the subject very quickly. I tried to bring him back to the subject by commenting, "Gee, sometimes it's scary to talk about people not being able to do things." He pretended not to have heard and started bouncing a ball.

The interview ended with his wanting me to play tennis and basketball with him. He was quite intent on playing a game, almost insisting on an answer. He showed a lot of longing and emotional hunger. I felt as though he wanted to take me home to be his friend.

Comments

Doug's physical and neurological functioning seemed intact. His mood conveyed an underlying sadness, longing, and depression, in contrast to the happy assertiveness one would expect of an 8-year-old. He projected an overall relatedness that was intense and emotionally hungry in style. There was a clear capacity for human relationships, but it had an affect-hungry quality to it rather than the sharing we would ordinarily expect in an 8-year-old. The affect system appeared organized but lacked depth and variety. I observed a general apprehension studded with preoccupations about guarding against future emergencies and fear of being hurt, robbed, and ill. I did not see a range of affects—from empathy and love to competitive anger, for example. Rather, the affect range was constricted around fearful concerns and some competitive feelings toward siblings.

In terms of developmental levels, it was clear that Doug could attend and engage, enter into two-way gestural communication (with some initial freezing), and construct representations or ideas. It was also evident that even at the gestural level, there were affective constrictions. At the representational level, we also see constrictions and some isolated islands of lack of differentiation, as will be described below.

There was competent age-appropriate thematic organization (though not content) except on the subject of his father's physical limitations, which provoked an abrupt switch in topic. Near the end of the interview, however, the organization loosened remarkably; although he kept to the topic, he seemed almost to be free-associating like an adult in psychoanalysis. His concern that his brother might find out what he was saying demonstrated a breakthrough of seemingly unrelated fantasy into his reality, an island of lack of representational differentiation. This breakthrough, together with his hungry style of relatedness, raises a question about the integrity of his personality structure. That this structure is below the age-appropriate level would be a hypothesis worth examining.

In terms of thematic depth, richness, and range, although I saw that this child was able to communicate a number of his concerns vividly, these concerns were few. That he was able to share what was on his mind is an important asset, yet he made no mention of school, mastery, friendships, or other common age-appropriate concerns, and, instead, was concerned with a limited number of highly emotional themes.

The thematic sequence gives us important clues to his conflicts. His concern with doing things right, followed by his worry that robbers might take his brother, fear of the future, and fear of bodily injury, dramatizes how close to the surface many of his conflicts are. The sequence shows him to be an emotionally hungry child who feels the need for more physical warmth and closeness from human beings, and who worries about how he can satisfy these needs.

My subjective feeling toward Doug was initially positive. I thought him an interesting and talkative child capable of making fairly good contact. I felt his warmth. Before long, however, I felt a sense of apprehension, thinking that this child was going to be very demanding; I was not sure that I wanted to get close to him. I thought, "This child wants more than I may want to give." My feelings ranged from being elated to feeling trapped. I had no noteworthy idiosyncratic fantasies during that hour.

CASE 2

Interview

Harold, a 7½-year-old, was in the waiting room with his mother when I first saw him. Most notable was his running back and forth in a seemingly provocative way, teasing his mother. When she insisted that he sit down for fear that he would break something, he sat fidgeting in a chair for about 30 seconds, then got up and started throwing a little ball that he had brought. He disregarded his mother's continuing commands that he return to his seat.

I introduced myself to Harold and he willingly came into the playroom, where he continued throwing his ball. Twice the ball came close to me, and my immediate subjective reaction concerned the degree to which Harold was aiming the ball at me. He spoke in a clear but nasal voice with a slight lisp. His gross motor coordination, which was amply displayed since he was continually in motion, seemed age-appropriate. Later on during the interview, when he showed me how he could make letters, I noted that his fine motor coordination seemed less than age-appropriate. His letters were indistinct; he often failed to close circles and missed many connections between loops and lines.

While moving around the room throwing his ball, Harold made good eye contact with me and kept coming to and fro in a playful manner, although he did not engage me in his ball-throwing game. He looked around the entire room and at the various toys. He quickly picked out a gun, threw the ball up, and pretended to shoot it. He commented, "This is fun," but again did not try to involve me. He continued to throw the ball and shoot it with the gun for a few minutes. Then he spotted some racing cars, which he instantly grabbed and started zooming along the floor, one car after the other. He seemed to lack the patience or capacity to roll them on their wheels, but rather shoved them almost as though to throw them, seeing which one would go farthest and fastest. Around this time I commented that he was interested in movement and speed as reflected in the cars and in his running around. Ignoring my comment, he continued to race the cars. He did not look in my direction while I was talking, nor did he respond, although he did talk to his cars, saying, "Speedo, speedo, you'll beat the other one."

He spotted ropes hanging from the drapes in the room and began pulling on them and spinning them around. I had to intercede for fear that he would pull the ropes off. With a flirtatious grin on his face, he taunted and teased me that he would not stop. After a while, however, he sensed that my patience was growing thin, and, when I told him to stop in a loud firm voice, he took three more seemingly playful swipes and then went back to zooming the racing cars. He then went over to a big Bobo doll in the corner of the room and began boxing with it, announcing, "I can beat up anyone, I am Superman." He was swinging at the Bobo in a somewhat chaotic fashion and I suggested, "Superman can do lots of things. What are all the things that you can do that are like Superman?" For the first time he chose to engage me. He said, "I'm strong, I can beat up all the kids at school. I can beat up my brother"(who is younger than he), and he continued hitting the Bobo. I commented that he seemed pleased by the fact that he could beat up all these people. He grinned, still hitting the Bobo. After this he found the gun again and started shooting at the Bobo, pretending the Bobo was the bad guy. This play began to have a somewhat more organized character as he hid behind a beanbag to shoot at the Bobo. Again, he did not involve me in the game or want me to become part of it.

At this point I began a running commentary on his play; one comment was that he was fighting with the bad guy. He said, "Yeah, I got to kill the bad guys." I wondered out loud who the special bad guys in his life were. He looked in my direction for a second and then grabbed the ball and started throwing it in my direction. I wondered out loud if he thought I was a bad guy. He looked away and started throwing the ball more frantically. I commented that sometimes bad guys can be scary. He then switched back to the racing cars and, still moving at a fairly frantic pace, began looking in my direction more frequently. He did not on his own, however, allow for any interactive game or communication with me.

The end of the interview was approaching, and I suggested that he might enjoy doing some drawing. He immediately took the crayons, pen, and pencil and starting throwing them at the Bobo as though they were knives. In response to my firmly structured suggestion, he agreed to sit down and draw something. First, he showed me how he makes letters at school. As indicated above, I noticed that his capacity to form letters was less than optimal for his age. When I suggested he draw a picture of his family, he rebelled against the idea and instead said that he was going to draw a forest, which became multicolored, disorganized circles. In response to questions about his family, he said that his mother was a good cook. With regard to his father, he said, "He hits me." He responded with silence when I asked him about his brother. When I asked whether he ever had any dreams, he shook his head to mean no. He may not have understood what I meant by dreams, even though I explained about seeing pictures when he closes his eyes. He ended the interview without any particular emotional reaction but was able to shake hands in response to my reaching out my hand.

Comments

Harold was a healthy, good-sized 7½-year-old. In terms of physical and neurological status, his gross motor coordination seemed quite appropriate. However, his fine motor coordination, as indicated by his inability to form certain letters, seemed below the age-appropriate level and raised some questions about his perceptual motor capacity. Moreover, he seemed to lack a capacity for focused concentration, as evidenced by his being in constant motion in both the waiting room and the playroom. With some effort on my part he could become focused, but was always easily distracted. Further, the capacity for developing organized themes, which he showed to some extent, was interfered with by his need to be in constant motion. He seemed reasonably intelligent in the way that he dealt with the playroom and developed his games. Although there was no special opportunity for seeing what his level of intelligence was, it did not appear to be outside age-appropriate norms.

Harold made human contact with me only through glances. Although the number of glances increased slightly toward the end of the interview, there was no deepening sense of relatedness. He made almost no attempt to involve me in his play or to communicate directly with me. It was as though I were just another object in the room of which he took note and was cautious. The only affective relatedness to me was around the theme of "the bad guys." It is possible that his constant activity may have been working against a more latent capacity for developing relatedness. With a child his age one would expect a deepening warmth and sense of relatedness in the context of a variety of affects and themes. With this child, however, the capacity for relatedness was not at the expected level.

His mood was stable throughout and could be described as one of wild excitement combined with some apprehension. The way he constantly moved around certainly had an excited quality to it; yet there was also the sense of apprehension, particularly when he was involved in the shooting game with the bad guys.

The main affects he showed were his concerns with competition, winning, and being powerful, along with some indication of fear. There was little expression of warmth, empathy, love, or real curiosity about what was available to him in the room, or available from communicating with me. When I wondered whether I was the bad guy, his anxiety was reflected in the way he quickly shifted activities and increased the activity level. This shift did not show a severe disruption; rather, it was a quickening of the pace of his already heightened activity level. He showed an ability to continue evolving the themes, however. Overall, particularly in terms of his range and types of affects, he seemed to be struggling with affective concerns below the $7\frac{1}{2}$-year-old level, where concern about power, competition, winning, losing, and fear of bad guys would be expected to dominate.

In spite of the immoderately high level of activity, Harold was able to show a capacity for small units of organized themes which hung together when reviewed in the perspective of the entire interview. That is, the themes of winning, aggression, competition, power, and eventually good guys and bad guys were presented in an organized fashion. It was notable, however, that these themes were presented in fragments or, one could say, that his dramas were divided into short and disconnected acts of very intense activity, in contrast both to acts that have continuity with each other and to acts that are longer, more leisurely, and thus more fully developed. Here again, it seemed that his activity level interfered with his ability to focus his concentration. There was some development of themes, but not the rich, deepening development that might be expected from a 7½-year-old. Harold kept the themes of power, competition, aggression, winning and losing, and good and bad guys at a fairly concrete, superficial level, revealing little about what was behind these concerns.

Developmentally, we see some attainment, but some compromises in all the early levels. Attention is fleeting; engagement is present but not deep or warm; two-way gestural communication is only intermittently present with some facial gestures, intermittent eye contact, and occasional verbal responses. Often, however, he ignored me and didn't close his gestural or verbal communication circles by responding to my comments with comments of his own. Yet, he was able, at times, to give realistic responses and deal with the larger reality and structure of the playroom, suggesting present, but highly constricted, representational capacities.

The sequence of his themes progressed from racing, winning and losing, and being Superman, to fighting with bad guys and protecting himself from the bad forces. The sequence reveals a series of concerns more at the 5- or 5½-year-old level, as indicated above; that is, concerns with power, aggression, size, and opposing forces trying to overwhelm him.

My initial subjective reactions concerned being hit by the ball that he was throwing somewhat wildly. After the initial danger seemed over, I hoped to develop a deeper and richer communication. When such communication did not occur, however, I felt disappointed that an empathic rapport could not be established with this child. I did feel some relief that he was able to respond to structure during the interview and that the chaotic and frenzied activity did not intensify but, rather, slowed down as he got to know me better.

CASE 3

Interview

As I entered the waiting room Joan, almost 6, was standing. She looked rather shy and did not speak. I suggested that she come into the playroom and she did. She was cute, well-built, and apparently well-coordinated in both her gross and fine motor actions. She walked in a firm, confident manner and later showed she was able to draw and do other fine motor activities successfully.

She came into the room cautiously, walking slowly at first and not saying anything. She went to the Bobo first, grabbed his red nose, and said that it was not supposed to stick out. There was a slightly nasal, lispy quality to her speech that diminished as the session went on. She seemed almost too relaxed and passive. She took no initiative to open a dialogue, nor did she explore much of the room. After a few minutes I broke the stillness by saying that she was free to play with anything or talk about anything she wished. I told her the rules of the playroom: we could not hurt each other or break anything. She immediately went over to the desk and began drawing.

She drew a picture of a little girl. What looked like a beard was, she told me, jewelry the girl was wearing. She then spontaneously told me that she was born here in Washington, and that her little sister thought that she was born here, too, but she was actually born in Long Island. Upon inquiry she told me that she meant her 4-year-old sister. She then started talking about her brother as though I knew all about him. As she elaborated I discovered that he was 8 years old and that he used to be in a special math class. She talked about math and science repetitiously, using the same few ideas again and again. Then she told me that she knew her teacher's first name, and smiled as though she knew something she was not supposed to know. She revealed that she did not like Sunday school and did not like to go because of having to leave her dog, Winnie. She made a joke about Winnie-the-Pooh and laughed. She seemed to be relaxed and enjoying herself at this time, about midway through the session.

She told me that she had a best friend. Joan was finishing a drawing of a big girl in a small house, the house just fitting around the girl. There was also a small car. I asked her to tell me more about the girl, but she told me about the house instead. She said that something was wrong with the chimney: the chimney was pink, and pink things can fall off. She appeared relaxed. I asked if she could tell me more about the girl and the chimney and the roof. She replied that the girl was Little Red Ridinghood and then she drew a picture of the wolf pretending to be grandmother.

At this point, immediately after she talked about the wolf pretending to be grandmother, she started inquiring about the mirrors on the wall (they were one-way observation windows) with some curiosity and suspiciousness. Although she had not shown a great deal of exploration on a motor level, staying mostly in one spot, she now acted curious and started walking around the room and looking at things. I commented that Little Red Ridinghood must have been scared and unsure about the wolf, must have felt uncertain seeing as how her grandmother could be a wolf. I continued, "Maybe you feel a little uncertain with all these mirrors in the room, being in a strange place, not knowing what's going to happen, just like Red Riding-hood."

She was silent after my comment. She tore off the sheet of paper that she was drawing on and seemed to become decidedly apprehensive in her own quiet way. She then went over to the black-board and asked me for some chalk. I told her that there was no chalk in the room and asked what she wanted to write. She said something about writing "yes" and "you." She was not clear, and I could only wonder whether the "yes" was to signify that I was right, that she was feeling uneasy.

The chalk being unavailable to her, I offered some alterna-tives. She seemed more suspicious and apprehensive, but even with this anxiety, she began to communicate more with me. She looked out the window, then noticed a policeman doll in the playroom. She took the doll and flirted with the idea of dropping it out the window. She became coy with me and wanted to know if it was all right to drop the doll. She then said that I had taken all this from her, referring to the play materials on the desk. She said, "These are all mine. I'm taking them home with me."

She started to play with the toilet, which was part of the dollhouse, and began sticking all the dolls into the toilet. She put one doll on the toilet and then put its head in the toilet. I made a comment about the doll going into the toilet headfirst. She put another girl doll on top of the doll on the toilet, and then tried to stick everyone in together. She seemed to become more relaxed as she was doing this, and she giggled. Then she tried to take the baby doll's diaper off. This was hard for her to do because the diaper was made of cello-phane. She wanted me to close my eyes as she hid the baby doll. Then I was to guess where it was. (At a number of points throughout the interview she had wanted me to guess what she was drawing, thinking, saying, or doing.) She then went over to the blocks and began building an incline. She showed me how it worked, and began talking about a science project at school.

As the end of the interview was near, I asked if she ever had any dreams (a question I frequently ask in such sessions). Openly and without hesitation, she told me the following dream. She said, "Me, Pam, and Michael were walking home from school and there were these witches. It was Halloween before we got home, and then we were eating dinner and the witches gave us this bread, which had poison, and father ate the bread and fell off his chair. And then it was morning and I woke up." I said, "That sounds like a scary dream." Without comment she took a block and put it under her dress near her vagina. Immediately afterward, again showing curiosity, she came over to me and asked what I was doing. She pointed at my notes and asked what I was writing there. With a knowing look she indicated to me that my writing made her uneasy, that she did not want anything down on paper.

She then told me about a 2-year-old boy who said that water did not scare him anymore. She went on to tell me about her interest in baking a cake, and then told me that once her mother had stolen Hanukkah money from her and her sister. She was able to acknowledge that she got mad at her mother, and she said that she never got the money back. Apparently her mother had confessed to her that she had in fact taken the money because she was short of shopping money. The session closed at this point.

Comments

It was clear that Joan's motor coordination was appropriately intact for a 6-year-old.

Her emotional tone, although basically one of shyness, embraced the capacity to evolve a relationship with the interviewer. In terms of relations, she demonstrated an appropriate capacity for attachment. The initial shyness evolved into openness with and relatedness to the interviewer. This relatedness was differentiated around the thematic material. That is, she was able to integrate a sense of interpersonal relatedness with the representational themes that she was developing. It was not clear whether her level of interpersonal relatedness was predominantly dyadic or triangular.

In terms of the style and development of affect, Joan was quietly cautious, seductive, guarded, suspicious, and apprehensive. There were mild signs of aggression in her coyness and teasing, and a blatant display of hostility mixed with joyful assertiveness when she stuffed all the dolls into the toilet. There was little expression of empathy, warmth, or love, which raises some question about her capacity for, or access to, these affects. She made the quick shifts characteristic of anxiety by showing apprehension and then curiosity (asking questions first about the mirrors and then about my notes). Although she experienced definite points of anxiety during the interview, it is important to note that this anxiety was not disorganizing, nor did it disrupt the interpersonal relatedness or the sequence of themes that were evolving. Interestingly, the first abrupt shift to curiosity (leading to questions about the mirrors) followed the themes of either houses or little girls being too big or small, chimneys, things falling off, and whether or not grandmother (the interviewer?) was a wolf in disguise. This sequence suggests anxiety about size, attachments or things falling off, and people tricking one another.

With regard to Joan's use of the space, she was quite passive and shy at first. Later on, however, she was able to expand and use the room and its objects to tell her story. Following the rules, she did not break or throw things. Nevertheless, she teased me with the policeman doll: "I'm going to throw him out. Will you let me?" This shows that she can readily internalize structure and is able to regulate herself reasonably well.

Turning to the category of thematic development, Joan showed an age-appropriate capacity to organize thematic material in a continuous and relevant way; that is, her themes were logically connected from the beginning to the end of the interview. She was somewhat repetitious, both in her themes of destruction, anger, and things falling off, and in her displays of coquettishness and seductiveness. Near the end of the interview concerns with aggression and death were made quite clear with the dream of witches poisoning her father, and there was a hint of a connection with feelings about her body as she held the block next to her genitals.

There was a certain depth and richness to the material she presented in terms of her ability to be in touch with her feelings. Although there may have been some walling off of feelings in the positive realm, she was in touch with a wide range of negative feelings. Expressing them made her somewhat anxious, but this anxiety did not overwhelm her and, in fact, allowed her to become more expansive.

Developmentally, she evidenced an ability to focus and engage, to use gestures and words intentionally (opening and closing circles of communication), to represent and elaborate a selected number of themes with complexity and detail, and to differentiate her representations to some degree. In terms of connecting and categorizing her ideas, there was a tendency to be a little fragmented and to focus on fantasy rather than balance fantasy a bit more with reality (e.g., more discussion of school, friends).

Some question remains about the age-appropriateness of the thematic material. Were her themes more appropriate for a younger child? There was little indication of repression during the session, and we do not know whether she has in fact reached the developmental point of intense triangular concerns, although hints of feelings toward her father are present. She might be involved with her own bodily integrity and concerns—particularly around aggression. We want to keep in mind such questions about age-appropriateness when taking a history from parents. We will also use possibly more playroom interviews to help answer these questions.

The final comment takes note of my subjective experience of

Joan. Throughout the interview I was aware of a conflict between wishing to provide more structure and watching to see what she would develop on her own. She was putting sort of a tense effort into clearly attempting to relate to me in a reasonably warm and somewhat open manner.

CASE 4

Interview

When I first saw Cathy she was standing, looking somewhat sad and frightened, and holding onto her mother in a shy, fearful manner. She did not look at me. Later, when it was her time to come into the interview room, she was in another playroom assiduously washing utensils. A female assistant was there with her. When I entered this scene, again she did not look at me although she knew it was time to come into the other room with me. I said to her, "We'll go into the other room," and she finished cleaning up and came with me easily enough. Cathy was nearly 6 years old and had excellent motor control over both gross and fine movements. As I noted later her speech was very clear and she was unusually verbal.

After coming into the playroom with me, her affective tone changed remarkably. She smiled broadly in a flirtatious way. She gave the Bobo a big punch with a joyous, playful expression. She wanted to know why it did not get back up. Then she explored the rest of the room in a rather calm and relaxed style, picking up and examining things. Then she quickly went over and set up the doll family and the chairs and table. Looking at the toilet, she said, "I can use this as a chair . . no, I've got to clean it." When I inquired about this, she said, "Well, there are germs and I've got to clean it." She did not, however, make any attempt to go to the room where she had been washing utensils.

She asked if her brother (whom I had also seen) had come in here, and then immediately went to punch the Bobo. I inquired if she liked to punch her brother, and she answered that it was exciting to fight. Then she said, "Okay, Bobo, you've had it." She said that the Bobo came up behind her and shoved her. She then began kicking and biting the Bobo and pushing its head back, describing her actions to me. She expressed some concern that the air might go out of it. When I commented that it seemed she did not want to hurt the Bobo too much, she agreed that was the case. Next she went to the rocking horse and said, "It's too little for me," indicating that she was now a big girl.

She then went around the room and asked how much time was left. I could not tell whether she wanted time to play or, on the contrary, wanted to leave soon. I was inclined to the latter interpretation, however, because of her very ambiguity. My impresson at this time was that her saying, "No, no, I want to play as long as I can because I'm having a good time," was the opposite of what she was feeling.

She began printing letters; she spelled S-O-X, then said, "I goofed," and scribbled all over the letters. This behavior seemed to represent some degree of organization and freedom, and yet disorganization at the same time. She asked if she could draw on the table. When I asked what she thought about that, she gave up. She then said, "My mother doesn't let me scribble on the table at home. We don't have much at home." I inquired about this and she said that her father brought paper to her, perhaps indicating that "daddy" was, in her view, the giving, nurturing figure.

She then discovered a salt container and began putting salt on the paper. She put some on her clothing and said, "This is my uniform at school. See how clean it is." Then, under the guise of making the paper clean, she began spilling salt all over it. Pouring out salt, she became very excited as it spilled all over the paper and the toy animals. I commented on her excitement and she said that her mother did not allow her to do that. She quickly went back to the salt, saying, "I think I'll eat some," and she tried to give some to the baby dolls. She put salt in a baby bottle and indicated that the dolls did not like it. She tried it herself and said, "I don't like it." She was also concerned about getting the salt in a small cut she had on her hand. Then she gave some salt to the toy hippo and pretended that he liked it.

She said she needed a spoon and wanted to go to the other playroom to get one. Since the door to the other room was locked, I suggested that we find something else she could use. She found a small dump truck for the purpose, easily adjusting to the fact that she could not have a spoon. She put salt on the crayons and was delighted with messing with the salt. She put salt on the rug, and I told her she should not because that made it difficult for the people cleaning the room. She tested the limits by first putting a little more salt on the rug and then putting some on the table.

I commented about the difference between here and home, that maybe she was concerned about the things that she could or could not do. I asked how she felt about the freedom she was experiencing here. She told me, "I throw things at home. I threw something at my mother." She then quickly said, "No, I didn't. I'm just making up a story." A moment later she said, "I kick Mother." Then added, "No, I don't. I'm just making up a story." I asked, "Would you like to kick Mother?" She said, "Yes, but I don't want to hurt her feelings." She then went back to the salt, pretending it was water, and began pouring it on the mother doll. She said the mother and a little girl were drowning in the water. Then she pulled them out, saying that they had jumped out. Next she put them in the washer and washed their hands.

She inquired about the time, and I asked how much more time she wanted. She said she wanted lots of time to play, which I again thought was an ambivalent response.

She said, "I hope Mark [her brother] stays out there"(in the waiting room). I asked if she was feeling at all anxious. She indicated that she was not, but she wanted to know if she and her mother were on time. She said she thought that they were late. She then indicated that she wanted to go into the other room where there were more toys and a sink.

At this point she went to the phone, which seemed to express a need to make an attachment either to Mark or her mother. I suggested that we could have a make-believe telephone conversation and talk to anyone she wished. She said, "You be John." She told me that John was her older brother who was in the Navy; he was stationed in a place where they make bombs and missiles. After telling me he was 18, she asked, "Is that too young to be a soldier?" Another question followed quickly: "How old are you?" Her affect was very flirtatious at this time and she came very close to me. I commented that she was curious about me and that maybe she could tell a story about me or about any thoughts that she had. She said, "You're a soldier and you make bombs. Let's pretend you're 18." I asked, "You mean, like your brother?" She then quickly went over and began hitting the Bobo. She said, "He makes me mad." I made a comment about her missing her brother since there seemed to be some relation between that possibility and punching the Bobo.

She asked if what she was telling me was going to be private. When I inquired about this, she said she would not want her mother to know. I asked what in particular she did not want her mother to know. She said, "Mother once threw a hamburger at Daddy. No, that's a story." Then when I inquired, she said, "Yes, but it missed Daddy." I asked her about her father and she said, "'Daddy has black hair. He's kind of dopey. He punches everyone once in a while." Then, "Oh, that's a story, too."

At the end of the interview I did some structuring by asking if anything scared her. She answered with slight excitement. "The doctor . . . giant monster . . . he goes 'ahh.' " She began jumping about, pretending to be a monster. I commented that maybe sometimes she liked to be the monster. She said yes, and indicated that she had terrible dreams of monsters; but again, the affect was one of joyous expansiveness. Then, telling me she was the monster, she came and punched me in the arm. She told me that she liked to make up stories, monster stories in particular. She began looking in some drawers and became very curious. The hour was up and I said that we would have to stop. She said she had more stories and I asked her to tell me the best one. The story again dealt with a monster and aggression. Her behavior near the end of the interview was both curious and seductive. Her looking in the drawers had the flavor of snooping—she pretended that no one knew what she was doing. She ended the session with a "good-bye" to me and a smile indicating some pleasure.

Comments

Cathy appeared to be physically intact and extraordinarily bright for her age. While she was able to regress freely and develop rich fantasies when given permission, she could also progress and respond to structure when it was indicated. Her verbal ability was unusually good.

Her overall emotional tone was one of joy and curiosity. She related in an intensely personal and intimate manner, constantly yet pleasantly insisting on my attention with her chatting and questions. Her relatedness showed a controlling quality as well as a seductive intrusiveness.

She demonstrated mostly joyous, explorative, excited affects of a wide age-appropriate range and depth during the course of the interview. As indicated, there was some show of diffuse anger, but in a playful way (with the Bobo doll), so that the anger seemed to be neutralized. Because of the expressive content of her anger—and yet little real display of anger—one may wonder about her tolerance for this affect. She showed some anxiety but was quite able to make transitions and continue her themes. Optimally, one might have expected a little more fearfulness and more negative affects; however, I gather from her references to her mother that she may show such feelings more with women than with men. Toward the end of the session, she became very flirtatious.

She took little time to begin exploring the entire playroom. Her play themes developed throughout the session and revealed a rich fantasy life that she had some control over. She revealed some conflicts, which she was able to deal with in a flexible way. She showed concern about doing well when she scribbled on a piece of paper, and wanted to know if she had goofed. She also seemed concerned about how organized or disorganized she was permitted to be, and looked for direct feedback from me. However, these hesitations were minor asides to her basically explorative, open, and fun-loving affective manner.

Developmentally, she was focused and engaged, very intentional in her gestures and expressive in her representational themes. Her ability to tie themes together and be logical with ideas suggested a solid capacity for representational differentiation.

Although Cathy's opening themes spoke of some conflict with messing and cleaning, she seemed to use the occasion of mother's absence to throw caution to the wind. It is possible that she feels freer with men than with women. She indicated feelings of both anger and fright toward her mother. Her feelings toward her father, who she said was sort of "dopey," were not clear. She revealed complicated feelings about her younger brother, showing some difficulty with her aggressive and fearful feelings related to his absence—she quickly shifted gears when discussions of her brother emerged.

In the beginning I felt quite relaxed with Cathy. Her demand for engagement by continuously looking at me and directing questions to me diminished as the interview went on, although I was always aware of her need to control. At one time I felt the conflict between how much I was to control the session and how much she was to control it. In the latter part of the interview, when she asked how old I was, I began feeling uneasy. The anxious feeling also occurred when she asked how much time we had, because I felt that she wanted to leave. In spite of the obvious interest and pleasure she was evidencing, there seemed to be a fear of her own excitement and both a worry about and capacity for ending the interaction. In general, she was able to arouse in me a variety of feelings around such issues as control, intrusiveness, and abandonment. I was impressed with both the variety and the continuity of her affects throughout the session. As the above comments suggest, her overall functioning seemed to be age-appropriate.

CASE 5

Interview

When I entered the waiting room to greet Steve, a 6½-year-old boy, he was crawling under the couch, making high-pitched gleeful sounds. His mother looked worried. All the magazines were strewn over the floor. When mother tried to comfort him, rubbing his back, he squirmed away and mother said, "He doesn't like to be touched." He came along easily, if not a bit overenthusiastically, into my office.

He tripped over his own feet, walking with a wide, somewhat unstable gait. He looked rigid and tight in his motor tone as he thumped around the room. His words were indistinct as he talked in a slightly hoarse voice, ran words together quickly, and mispronounced many sounds. Yet he was understandable. His fine motor coordination was quite clumsy as he quickly went searching through the toy closet, dropping small items and having difficulty manipulating the smaller, finer toys. Later he had difficulty in drawing circles and squares, etc.

He made fleeting, mildly impersonal contact with me through a quick glance and immediately thereafter went to the toys. A frantic quality quickly emerged as he tossed all the toys on the floor in a disorganized manner. He then kept asking me to name each toy and other objects in the room. When I commented on his "interest in knowing names of things," he again made fleeting eye contact and kept asking me to name items.

Often, he didn't respond to my gestures or words with gestures or words of his own. Only about 40% of the time did he seem tuned in and responsive.

He kept moving, at times running, around the room, looking excited, occasionally tripping, momentarily looking confused, and then would become excited again.

This pattern went on for about 10 minutes. He then came across a stick and, with a gleeful look, repetitively banged it against a chair. He then jumped on some crayons that I had spilled on the floor, and, taking a policeman doll, he began banging it on the floor, saying "Bad boy, bad boy." He momentarily looked "blank" and began rocking back and forth while sitting on the floor.

He then looked at me and asked, "Do you have any candy?" I commented that he wanted me to give him some candy, and he said "yes" and then started to throw a sponge ball at me, not stopping until I physically restrained him. He then said, "I want that horse" (a rubber play horse).

Nearing the end of the interview, I asked him about his parents, school, dreams, etc., and he only answered with regard to school, talking about "hitting kids" and "being bad." He named some children, but would not elaborate.

He left the interview still quite active, with a fleeting glance.

Comments

There were indications of uneven maturation as evidenced by a possible overreactivity to touch, difficulties with gross and fine motor coordination, difficulty comprehending or focusing on my gestures and words, hoarse and indistinct speech, and difficulty with modulating his activity level and impulses. There was also a perseverative quality to his questions of "What's this?" etc., and a ritualistic quality to some activities such as banging. In addition, there was a brief episode of rocking. All these observations raise questions about physical-neurological compromises.

His mood vacillated between undifferentiated excitement and an indifferent quality. He related to me but only fleetingly and with little depth. Relatedness was therefore also below age expectations. There was little of the age-appropriate range of affects of modulation (e.g., only undifferentiated excitement). Anxiety may be inferred in relation to the loss of relatedness (i.e., blank look), rocking, and the impulsiveness (e.g., throwing a ball at me) that occurred after the "bad boy" theme and request for candy.

The interview suggested that anxiety is disruptive to an already vulnerable integrative capacity and may be experienced at the most primitive level of somatic disorganization.

Developmentally, he evidenced compromises of a marked nature at all levels. Attention and engagement were intermittent and unstable. Two-way gestural communication and the overall ability to be intentional were also only partially established. There were some representational capacities, but they were only fleetingly present and not used as a predominant mode of communicating. He did show a few islands of differentiated representational capacity when he was logical in asking me for candy.

Thematic concerns were communicated in the following sequence: aggressiveness, loss of control, being a "bad boy," disorganization, hunger, anger. They reflected islands of cohesive thematic interests. Organization, range, and depth were all significantly below age expectations. By age 6½, cohesive, rich themes would be expected. There were no highly "bizarre" themes, however.

My subjective reactions vacillated between apprehension about his impulsiveness, lack of involvement, and some relief at the fleeting eye contact, indicating a potential for involvement.

CASE 6

Interview

David entered the interview room with a relaxed though somewhat clumsy gait. He was talking freely in a friendly way and his facial expression was relaxed. As the session progressed, he showed good gross and fine motor coordination and good modulation of his activity level. His contact with me was warm and friendly. He took in the entire room and was quite curious and exploratory in a reasonably systematic yet spontaneous and relaxed way. In short, in terms of his initial orientation to me and the room, he behaved quite up to the optimal expectations for his age of 5½ years.

He went to the racing cars first and told me that a tire was broken. Then he went around to all the toys, picking up and examining each one. He put on a cowboy hat, which fell off. He then began playing with the dolls and identified a father, mother, and son doll on his own. He said, "Hey, these things are puppets," and began playing with them. He talked about the mother doll sending some of the puppets to another part of the room. He went over to the gun and told me that it was broken (because he could not work it). He then told me that the cars did not run well, but played with them for a while. He developed a slight theme with the cars and got them going all over the place.

All this time David was friendly, but then, in the context of the car game, he showed me that he knew karate. He informed me that the son (doll) was having to take care of the daddy (doll) because the daddy's car had broken down. When I asked him whether the son had a better car, he got the son and father puppets and developed an elaborate story about the son's wanting to karate chop the father because the son could not get enough Coke to drink. The son and father got into a fight with the son trying to kill the father. Then the father gave the son a lecture, after which the son beat up the mother, saying, "I want a Coke." Finally the son got hurt and the mother kissed him and said, "You were a bad boy." The story ended with the son lying face down. This story lasted for about 15 minutes and was related very expressively, with David doing the talking for all parties. I was watchful, occasionally commenting in order to follow up on themes.

Soon after David finished this elaborate theme with the son beating up the father in the mother's presence, he wanted to go back to the other room. My own associations at this point were that, having had his catharsis, he now wanted to get away from the scene of the action. I asked about his wish to leave and told him he could return to the other room later. He then quickly picked up some animals and wanted to know what I was writing. He picked up another animal and said that it was a mother rabbit, a theme he stayed with for a while without actually developing it. He seemed to be resting while comforting himself with the mother rabbit. I inquired indirectly about the earlier scene by wondering if he was resting and relaxing from all that went on. He told me that when he gets angry he throws things and karate chops his brother. He said this happens when he does not get to go outside. He then went back to the dolls, further developing the theme of aggression. He talked about the dolls liking each other, but he placed them face down.

We were now near the end of the session. I asked about

mother and he said, "Very nice." He picked up a car and then an animal, and said about the latter, "This is a dinosaur." I asked him about father and he said, "I don't know. I don't know anything about him, but I know he is very nice—he is a lawyer." Then he came back to his mother, saying, "Don't know about Mommy." Then he started talking about a little girl named Mary Lou who was very nice. He then commented that there were not as many toys here as in the other room and started telling me about a friend called Robbie "who is a mean person who throws things." I asked about his sister; he said that she was nice and that his brother was very nice. I asked if he had any dreams, and he told me he had a dream about Winnie-the-Pooh doing something naughty and awakening the Scottie puppy. He ended the interview in a relaxed fashion without any particular affective expression.

Comments

David appeared to have age-appropriate sensory and motor capacities, good receptive language, and reasonably clear speech. He was personable in manner, maintaining good contact throughout the interview. He demonstrated an overall quality of curiosity and warmth, and showed capacities for pleasure and enjoyment as well. He related to the interviewer with interest but without any deepening of affect. He did not ask questions but developed a particularly rich theme and a few subthemes largely on his own.

He demonstrated a rich variety of age-appropriate emotions, but his main concerns were with anger, competition, and with not getting enough feeding. When he got anxious and wanted to leave after the Oedipal-type family drama was elaborated, he was quickly able to shift his attention to other things. There was some suggestion that his drama of conflict and anger was fueled by an early concern with not getting enough (i.e., "Coke"). In addition, there are suggestions that he doesn't see a clear way to resolve his need to get more. The drama ends with the boy face down; mother is associated with a dinosaur and the mother rabbit is not presented as a "filling up" experience.

He was both explorative and organized in the playroom. He dealt with themes of anger by, in part, displacing them into games. Yet he showed that he understood the limits of the playroom.

Developmentally, he evidenced solid mastery of all levels. He was focused and engaged, capable of intentional two-way gestural communication, and able to elaborate and differentiate a rich representational drama.

David developed a cohesive and organized theme focusing

on the family struggle and fighting with father. Most impressive was the way he played the theme out by modulating the emotions and affects of each party. The theme of family aggression and conflict dominated the session; no equally rich thematic development occurred around his pleasurable or dependent pursuits except in reference to wanting a Coke from his parents.

Subjectively, I felt more intellectually than emotionally "filled-up." I felt as David did. Perhaps the complex Oedipal drama doesn't fill either of us up.

As suggested above, David's functioning is in the age-appropriate range.

CASE 7

Interview

Joey was a trifle small for his age of 5¼ years, and his voice was slightly nasal or lispy. He was sucking his thumb and holding onto his mother when I first met him. He announced, "I won't let her go," and said to her, "I'm going with you." His mother cajoled him, attempted to bribe and manipulate him in various ways, but could not get him to go into the playroom without her.

Although apprehensive, he moved slowly and evenly, and appeared to have good gross and fine motor coordination. He avoided eye contact with me, looking instead at his mother as if to deny my presence. Anxious though he seemed, there was a grin on his face when engaged in the verbal battle with mother about whether she would stay in the playroom with him. He did explore the playroom to an extent, but stayed close to mother. She seemed reluctant to give him directions.

As the session went on he relaxed somewhat, talking with me and glancing at me from time to time. Throughout, however, the basic and major tie was to mother. It was difficult to assess the degree to which he was indeed frightened and the degree to which he was receiving gratification from manipulating his mother. Interestingly, the mother tried in numerous ways to get him to stay on his own, including telling him later in the interview that she "had to go to the bathroom or I'll make in my pants." To this he responded that he would accompany her and stand outside the bathroom.

Once in the playroom with mother, he sat on the Bobo and pulled its nose, announcing, "I'm going to let the air out." He looked at me to see if I was angry and then proceeded to let the air out. After playing with the Bobo he said he wanted to draw. He drew and tried to write his name. He then moved on to lining up some play animals and announced to me that the giraffe was the biggest one. He then became concerned about the window being open and wanted to close it. I asked him about that and his response was to threaten to throw one of the animals out of the window. Overall, his manner was characterized by a mildly provocative, controlling quality with brief shifts to coy pleasure and occasional displays of apprehension.

He went to the toy dog and announced that it was the smallest animal. I asked how he thought the dog felt being the smallest, and, after some deliberation, he said, "They will eat him up." When I said, "That must be pretty scary," he went over and began bouncing the ball. He proceeded to pick up a horse and then figures of a cowboy and an Indian. He found a gun which he pointed at his mother, and then became angry, saying, "Why doesn't it work? Where's the bullet? It's lost." He then became involved with the fireman and the cowboy and tried on their hats. He announced that the hats were both too small, and then said that one was too big and one was too small. He then wanted to know if there was a television set in the room. I said there was none and asked about his interest in TV. He discussed with me the possibility of his putting on a TV show. Then he picked up the man puppet and, putting it near his mother's face, said, "He is crying." Shortly after that he went out of the room with mother, accompanying her to the bathroom, as referred to above.

By the time they returned the interview was almost over, and I began to structure the final moments. I asked, "If you could have three wishes, what would they be?" He said for the first wish he would want nothing; for the second wish, he said, "I want a real gun with real bullets to shoot people—only bad people, but people who fight with me." I inquired about people who fight with him and he told me about his friend Jimmy: "He beats me up." For the third wish, he first wanted a basketball and then decided on a Bobo doll because he liked hitting the Bobo.

Interestingly, it was during this phase of the interview, when I was asking specific questions, that I felt he was more relaxed with me. I asked if he ever had dreams. It was unclear whether what he proceeded to tell me were real dreams, pieces of TV shows that he had watched, or daydreams. Nevertheless, he reported something about TV shows and a witch and two small children who sneak up on the witch's house. There was someone in the house with a long mustache and a beard. He did not go on. I proceeded by asking about any scary dreams, and he told me, "We all saw a movie and my brother threw up in the toilet. My brother had to sleep with Mommy in the same room." He also told how he had bad dreams after watching the movie and was scared that he was going to be locked in somewhere. During this recital he kept looking at his mother. I then asked if he had any questions for me. He proceeded to bring me a dead insect that he had found and told me a little dog had scared the insect. He then stood up next to his mother, took the gun out, and said, "Is time up?" I said that it was and ended our session.

Comments

Although small for his age, Joey seemed to be neurologically sound, with his gross and fine motor coordination, perceptual motor ability, and receptive and expressive language all apparently intact. His overall mood was one of apprehension. Predominant affects demonstrated in the interview were the tendency to cling, apprehension, and anger—although there was a facade of playful and pleasurable manipulativeness around the issue of control. He needed to keep mother with him. The anxiety he manifested seemed to center on separation and aggression. When he related to me, the quality was mostly of apprehension. As indicated, he responded better when I structured things for him with questions, which enabled him to relate to me somewhat warmly. Even then, however, there was only minimal affective depth and his tone was one of reluctance. For the most part, his was a superficial yet distinctly human involvement with the interviewer. Control, provocativeness (teasing), and the use of distance characterized his style of relatedness.

He did not deal with the entire playroom but tended to stay in one area, usually near mother. Nor did he develop cohesive themes, but rather moved from one idea or thing to another. These bits and pieces had little richness. In a limited way he was able to dramatize some of his conflicts around the issues of aggression, his tie to mother, his feeling small, and his experience of danger. He showed some concerns about being engulfed (e.g., the little dog being eaten up) and about injury (e.g., shooting). He demonstrated a dependency on mother which seemed below an age-appropriate level. His mother seemed to be unable to help him resolve this attachment and in some respects played into his hands.

Developmentally, he evidenced an ability to focus and engage and use intentional gestural communication. He could also represent and differentiate experience. But his representations tended to be fragmented, constricted, and unable to fully assist him in creating an internal sense of security that would help him separate from mother. Therefore, while partially differentiated, he operated for the most part in a representationally fragmented and constricted manner.

My initial subjective feeling was one of discomfort at his unwillingness to separate from mother. However, I soon found myself calmly enjoying the scene of mother's struggles with him, feeling relieved that I was not in her place. I was not in touch with any fantasies during the session, which, on the whole, I found neither difficult nor pleasurable.

As this summary suggests, Joey was functioning below age expectations for a 5¼-year-old in almost all the areas of functioning.

CASE 8

Interview

Warren was a very handsome 9¾-year-old youngster, with a funny hat and a big jacket, looking "cool" and well dressed. It looked like very well planned casualness. As he sat down, he had a kind of "Don't hassle me" look, as though he were saying, "I'll confess to anything if you just don't hassle me." I asked him how I could help and he said, "I guess getting my schoolwork done is the main problem." He was then able to begin elaborating on this theme.

In those first few minutes, he established that he could be warm and engaging, that his mood was even, that he had good focus and concentration and good impulse control, and that he was articulate and organized and understood my comments. A number of his basic personality functions, such as the ability to separate reality from fantasy, were all quickly established as age-appropriate.

Even in the first few seconds, however, he clued me in to the special issues for him, with his "Don't hassle me, I'll confess. I'm guilty of all kinds of sins and misdemeanors" look. Also, together with that "Don't hassle me, I'll confess" sort of look, there was a look of sadness in his eyes and of being overwhelmed at times. He elaborated, "Okay, getting into my schoolwork, getting it done is the problem. There's too much work. I try, but I can't always get it done, particularly the long assignments. Particularly, you know, with writing. I need some new inventions to make life easier (in the twenty-first century). Something that would help me with writing, and that stuff."

As I summarized what he said, he went on, "I do my best, but like I forget my spelling book and things like that." Then he revealed the situations (his tale) that undermine his best efforts. He told me many stories about forgetting. The details were always vague. As he talked, the level of tension increased. He was digging himself into a hole as he was gradually becoming aware that his seemingly logical explanations didn't quite fit together.

During this time, I tried to be especially supportive rather than challenging to help him talk about what happens, how he forgets his books or his homework assignments or the time of his class. More of his sadness came through. He became even more vague as I followed his story. At the same time he continued to be warmly engaged. His concentration, impulse control, and sense of connectedness remained quite good even when he was feeling tense and sad.

He then switched from the schoolwork to friends. He told me about a second grader who's a year younger and lives on his block. He knows this child "always lies." He likes him but he doesn't like his lying. Then there's this other boy at school and "other friends," but "they're not always available (in fact), often not available, but it's no big deal." He said repeatedly, "no big deal, I don't really care." He went out of his way to suggest, "Let's keep it cool, let's keep it low-key, not get too upset with all this."

I empathized that "It's important for things not to bother you too much, for things not to be a big deal, that you like to keep things in perspective." He said, "Yeah, that's kind of my life's philosophy, keep things mellow, and cool, in perspective."

I asked him how that played out in the family. He said, "It can get tense with Mom and Dad, but it's okay. My older sister gets too angry, and my brother tricks too much. My younger sister is always whining. Don't like her always getting me into trouble." He went over the family members pretty quickly. He was only prepared to elaborate on the one sibling who got him into trouble.

He didn't want to talk about his parents, or how he would like them to change. He wanted to "stay away from that. I would get too spoiled if they were too calm."

With the focus on keeping things "calm," I wondered how he best does that. He then got into the theme of just "forgetting things," and how "forgetting stuff" is his biggest problem at school. I said, "Let's look at the steps" of how he manages to forget. As we were looking at the steps, he again went through a series of examples where he "just forgets stuff," however hard he tries to remember. Then he described how it just "builds up and builds up," and sometimes he just feels like "chucking it over my shoulder." I said, "I think you just put your finger on the key, 'chucking it over your shoulder.' " He then described an image of "shit—building up, and building up, and piling up [on him.] And then just say 'chuck it!' " He smiled, and the tense, depressed, sad look lifted. The smile grew bigger as he talked about "chucking it," and the relief of "just forgetting it all."

I wondered why he doesn't like to face certain things, when it gets "too hot," and instead he likes to just "chuck it," and why he enjoys "chucking" so much. He said, "I just want to get away."

I wondered if he does that with feelings. He clarified, "You mean I get embarrassed about certain feelings and I also push feelings away?" I nodded and he said, "I don't like to get angry." I wondered, "Things get you angry, even though you like to be calm." He said, "Sort of. Well, teachers at school, they favor the girls." He then gave an example of playing soccer, and how the teachers were more protective toward the girls. "They don't let the boys beat the girls as much as they could. I was mad."

I wondered if that happened in other settings too. He said, "At home, Mom favors my 12-year-old sister, who likes to boss me." He described how his sister bosses him, and how his mom sides with his sister. He saw an alliance between the two of them, as though he had two moms—too much for him to cope with.

Dad, he said, is more even, "But he's away a lot." He described how he doesn't see his potential male ally in the family helping him with "these two women." Then he said in his characteristic fashion, "But no big deal," downplaying his feelings. I commented that I could tell "how he would rather chuck these feelings over his shoulder."

We then talked about how he might pay attention in his own way to the feeling of wanting to "chuck it." When he wants to say it's "no big deal," is perhaps the time to focus on what it is that he wants to "chuck." At least then if he is going to chuck it, it will be an intentional decision.

As the session came to a close, I sensed his sadness building up a little. He seemed to want to continue.

Comments

Warren's basic personality functions of reality testing, impulse control, relatedness, and concentration all appeared age-appropriate. I was impressed with the amount of denial and avoidance he needed to use to deal with emotional issues that were difficult for him. I was also impressed with the underlying sadness. He didn't show much anger, but there were hints of anger connected to the sadness.

At the end of the interview, I did some academic kinds of things with him (e.g., recalling numbers forward and backward, copying shapes and recalling shapes). His auditory and visual/spatial memory for the short, mechanical tasks was not so developed as his general intelligence. The mechanical, rote memory side of life is, therefore, probably very hard for him, compared with his reasoning and abstracting ability. He tried to avoid these tasks with me and no doubt avoids them even more in his competitive private school.

I was also impressed that during the latter part of the interview, he did some therapeutic work. He was figuring out why he "chucked" things. He was also able to begin explaining a feeling of anger and unfairness with regard to his sister.

Throughout the interview, he related well and had an even mood, but evidenced only a narrow range of affects and themes. There was denial of anger and an underlying sadness. His "chuck it, keep calm" defense was a type of "What, me? Who, me? Where did it all go?" He was also obviously very charming and liked to manipulate his way out of conflict. I had no doubt that part of his openness with me was in this vein. Yet I also felt that as his sadness and anger were reached, he would become more genuine. My subjective reaction was one of pleasure and relaxation. Warren was very likable, a sign of his potential for warmth and his ability to charm others, especially when he was anxious.

CASE 9

Interview

Ten-year-old Danny came into the office on his own and was extremely friendly, almost as if he had known me for many, many years. He had a big smile, sat down right away, looked me in the eyes, and radiated warmth. He started chatting about his life, mostly about school. His concentration and focus were good as he looked at me, staying on the subject of school, and sitting in one spot for most of the session, except for when he switched from the chair to the floor, sitting with his legs crossed like an Indian chief. His impulse control was excellent as he followed the implicit rules of the playroom, talking rather than throwing things or breaking things. His mood was on the excitable side, with a great deal of anxiety and sense of exasperation about things that weren't going exactly his way. There was more a "how dare they do this to me" quality than a sense of sadness, depression, or emptiness. He evidenced a mixture of outrage, worry, anxiety, impatience, and a flighty hyperness and tension.

As he sat down, with a big smile, he immediately said, as though he had been primed by his mother or had been waiting to see a psychiatrist for many years, "I have too many enemies in school. I don't know what to do about them. They tease me." When I inquired in what way they tease him, he said, "They talk behind my back, spreading rumors about me." He readily gave an example, saying, "One time I came in with new sneakers on and was very proud of them and someone started making fun of the style, saying they looked yucky. Then that person started giggling with the other kids behind my back. Then they spread rumors. I can't figure out exactly what they were."

He then went on listing other things that embarrassed him. "I'm sort of between toy cars and big-kid stuff, not quite there yet. One time I hit another kid, just sort of friendly, not to really hurt him, but he was getting mean and I sort of pushed him a little bit and then his friends all became my enemies."

"What I really need are friends I can count on, but there's this kid I read with—he's real cool and I worry about losing friends to him. Every time I have someone I think I can count on he seems to make friends with them and take them away from me."

I inquired as to how he felt about this state of affairs and he said, "I feel so angry. I'm enraged. I get this feeling in my head, it goes to my chest. I want to cry. I feel tight. It's not just a physical feeling, it's like I'm upset and I want to cry and I feel too emotional and yet I also feel like my heart isn't working right."

I inquired further about what the feelings were like and he said, "I feel so mad sometimes I feel so mad I get sad." I wondered about the difference between the sad feeling and feeling sort of frenzied, overwhelmed, and angry, and he said, "Well, I feel sad when my middle brother acts up, when we can't go out, like if we're supposed to go to the movies or something on a nasty day, or sometimes, even worse, my little brother, who tends to be the aggressive one in the family, if he has been bad we all get punished for him. Then I feel disappointed. But that's different from when I feel angry and cornered by one of the kids at school."

As I summarized some of the feelings he was telling me about— how he feels disappointed and other times he feels cornered, overwhelmed, and angry—he smiled. I commented on his pleasure in my comment and he said, "Well, I may be smiling but actually when these situations happen I feel furious inside." He went on, "Often, I try to put on a nice face. I smile in class; I smile at other kids. I want to be friendly, but I might be feeling cornered and overwhelmed and really enraged at them inside but I keep those thoughts private." I wondered that he must feel it is best to keep all his feelings private and he said, "If people would know how angry and furious I get, no one would be my friend." I said, "No one?" He said, "No one." I wondered whether these were just people at school or even his family or the world in general and he said, "Well, the only one who might be my friend would be my little brother because he's mean and he might understand how mean I feel. But my mother and father don't like me to be angry or mean, although I've seen my mother be mean to me—she has quite a temper—she can yell and scream. And certainly the teachers and the kids at school, they would probably, some of them would just start teasing me and I couldn't take that. And I think the teacher thinks of me as a nice boy and kind of her pet and she wouldn't like it either."

I commented on his dilemma. He then went on to say, "After a fight when Warren gets other kids after me and they kind of pick on me, I often feel very alone. I feel like I'll never have a friend again. I feel like crying. It's an empty feeling inside me. I feel very alone." When I commented that this "alone" feeling seems to be very upsetting and very painful, he went on to say, "I hate that feeling. It's the feeling I dread the most, to have no friends." He further elaborated, "At home, my mother tends to be very busy, often grading papers and things for school. My father works hard. I hate my two brothers. I feel very much alone some of the time. I have some kids around the block I could play with but I feel like sometimes there's no one I can be close to. Other times I might like my mother and we might be really talking."

He then went on to associate, quite on his own, about how angry he feels. "I can't stand it when I get cornered and then people aren't proud of me. I get so mad." (He was hinting at a relationship between this part of himself that no one but his little brother can understand, his mean side, and this lonely feeling where he feels he can't be close to anyone—hinting perhaps that his meanness and embarrassment over it makes him feel very much alone.)

It was then getting near the end of the session and I suggested that he might like to draw a picture. He drew a picture of a house with lots of detail, including windows and doors. There were clouds and trees around it, but there were no people. It was a detailed house without life or richness to it. He said, "I added a clubhouse to the house for friends. I can get away to the clubhouse, especially to get away from my dad because he bugs me, wanting me to study harder and get better grades. My mom bugs me too and my two brothers, I really need to get away from them. But Dad screams the most, he really makes me feel like I can't think when he screams so loud."

"My mother bears down on me, not screaming like my father does, but she just creates pressure. I don't know what to do to get away from her. I have no peace. Even the housekeeper bugs me."

I empathized with his dilemma, that he likes to have lots of friends and doesn't like to feel alone. He often wants to be in the middle of things, but at the same time people bug him and he wants to be back in the clubhouse all by himself (even though it's a clubhouse for friends). At this point he gave a big smile and said, "You seem to know how I feel. I can't stand it when anyone else is getting attention other than me. I mean, I get A's and I have the best ideas and I can sing and I'm a better musician than a lot of the kids, but I don't get the credit in school. I mean I should be the most popular kid but I'm not, Warren is, and he seems to have it in for me. He always wants to put me down. And I don't know what I could do to win out over the other kids." He then went on to describe how, "Even though I can do everything better than everyone else, I get confused easily, and I get real mad—my thoughts don't seem to work."

Comments

The impression at the end of this first interview was that Danny was a youngster who could attend and engage very warmly. He was capable of nice give-and-take communication, with appropriate gestures. He used ideas (representational) to communicate his feelings and thoughts in an organized and intentional way. He was obviously quite verbal and very bright. It was also evident, however, that he could easily get overloaded and feel fragmented and that, in interacting with others, he was very sensitive to every subtle emotional nuance. When he got overloaded he would feel fragmented and disorganized ("like a thousand thoughts all around me").

His mood was intense and at times frenzied. He evidenced lots of affects, mostly around anxiety over competition and neediness and fear of humiliation and loss. Themes were represented and sometimes organized, but they could also become fragmented. There were some indications that he had some conflicts between his desire to be the middle of everything, the ease with which he became overwhelmed, and the difficulties he had with dealing with certain basic wishes and affects having to do with anger and competition, as well as loss and disappointment. While he was engaged, attentive, and related interactively in gestures as well as concepts and words, he was limited in his ability to apply these capacities to certain realms of emotion. The emotions having to do with competition, anger, and loss were especially difficult for him. The implications of his conflict between his wish to be the center of everything and his fears of assertiveness and competition for his emerging sexual identity were not clear at this point. He didn't have close male friendships or comfortable role models and felt his father to be distant and critical. At times, he could feel close to his mother. This would be an important area to explore in a subsequent interview.

He evidenced a marked constriction in the flexibility of his personality, even though, for the most part, he had mastered aspects of engagement, two-way communication, using ideas to label and conceptualize emotions, and being able to organize emotions into categories. In this last capacity, however, when he was anxious, he lost this ability and felt overwhelmed and confused. He repeatedly reexperienced feeling overwhelmed and confused. In addition, when anxious, he quickly felt that he was treated unfairly by "enemies" (an all-or-nothing quality), rather than being able to see competition as an integral part of complex relationship patterns. He was unable to maintain a broad range of affects and also unable to consider all possibilities for other people's actions. Inflexibly he replayed the same "drama" ("They are my enemies") over and over. My subjective reaction was to feel a bit overloaded, much like Danny did, and at times not very drawn into the seemingly dramatic content.

In general, he was at age expectations in some categories (relating, organization of themes), but was below age expectations in others (mood, affects, anxiety, and thematic range and content).

CASE 10

Interview

Alice was a small, thin, intense-looking 7-year-old girl. She came into the office quickly, sat down, and stared silently. Her eyes looked tense and expectant. She seemed overloaded with feeling. She didn't go to the toys or begin talking or gesturing. There was, however, a sense of relatedness. I asked how I could be of help. She said, "Well, I'm not sure. I don't know." I wondered, "Is it sometimes hard to figure out what to say in new situations? Do you sometimes feel shy in new situations?" She said, "No, I'm actually not very shy." I said, "Oh, you tend to be more outgoing?" and she said, "Sometimes." She then told me about her best friend at school who is a person with whom she feels comfortable and very outgoing. They like to "play stuff together. She is my best friend."

As she was talking about this girl (she also mentioned that she has some other friends, but this is her "one main best friend"), I noticed that she was focused, related, and engaged, that she had energy, and that her thinking was organized. For example, she related details about her friend and school, giving examples of what they do together. She told of a game they play with dolls. She was able to explain that her friend "really likes that game; I like it, but not as much as her."

Initially, I was impressed with her ability to relate and reason, including comparing how much she and her friend like the doll game.

She went on to talk about school and other friends and told me she hates her current teacher, who yells at the kids and is kind of a "witch." She went from the teacher to her parents and how her "Mommy and Daddy" are mostly nice, but sometimes "they yell too much and Daddy can yell more than Mommy, but Mommy can yell a lot," and she doesn't like that at all and "it is upsetting." When they yell, she feels "very sad" and wishes she "was never born and I want to run away."

From there we went to talking about her brother who is older (he's 10) and "he likes to fight with me a lot." She wants to "wring his neck" when he is picking on her. He will punch her in the stomach and they'll mix it up and get each other into hot water.

She then mentioned that she likes her cats better than her brother. She "loves" to play with them. "The cats," she said, "can do all kinds of interesting things." When I asked her what sort of things, she said, with a matter-of-fact expression, that the cats can communicate with her. "They talk to me." She added that only she could understand and talk to the cats. "When they go 'meow, meow,' Mommy and Daddy would hear it just as 'meow,' but the cat is actually talking to me, telling me about what I want to do." "I also talk to the cats and they understand, like 'Go get me that,' and 'Go find a bird outside.' The cats do the things I say." She was discriminating about what the cats could and couldn't do. (I wondered if she often told the cats to do things that cats naturally do anyway to confirm her own ideas.)

After she finished telling me about the cats, I asked her if there were other kinds of experiences where she could do something that other people couldn't do. She looked at me and said, "What do you mean?" I said, "Are there other things that happen to you or that you can do that other people wouldn't know about?" She said, "Oh yes," and she proceeded to tell me about "voices." "They tell me nice things and bad things." If she is upset with her parents or her brother they might comfort her and tell her ways of getting even with her brother. They also tell her to "jump off the house." I asked her how she felt when the voices said these kinds of things like telling her to jump off the top of the attic. She said, "Well, they just say it once, and I don't want to do these things, so it doesn't scare me because I know they can't make me do it." It was important to her that "the voices just come and go; they aren't there always." Her affect was sort of matter-of-fact as she related these experiences. But she did add, "They are more of a pain than they are a help," and "I wish they weren't there. It has been getting a little less recently."

The cats and the voices had started in the last 6 to 8 months. I asked her where she thought the voices came from. She talked about a distant planet, like Earth. There were some beings there that were talking to her and sending her messages. I asked her if the planet had a name, and she thought for a second and said, "Apple." (I had the impression that she invented the name at that moment.) She didn't seem to have a complex system worked out and said that she would rather "they left her alone," that they would "go away."

She told me "the voices" also talk to her best friend (not the cats, just the voices). She further elaborated that when she gets really mad at her brother and wants to beat him up and gets sad and wishes she were never born, the voices will comfort her. We talked about strong feelings and how the voices and cats sometimes help with these. I wondered which feelings were hardest. She felt her parents' fighting scared her and that they either fought or "don't talk to each other." She sometimes felt "alone." She didn't feel there was any particularly strong feeling going on just before the voices or cats started talking to her. As the interview drew to a close, she reiterated that she wished the voices would go away.

Comments

Alice was a small, very attractive 7-year-old with good gross motor coordination. I didn't get a chance to observe her fine motor skills. She spoke clearly and articulately with full, complex sentences. She seemed to have good receptive and expressive language skills. Her mood was even and intense. While her content suggested escapist and depressive themes, her overall mood was not lethargic or depressive in nature. She related very warmly and was quite engaged and open. Initially, she showed some cautiousness and even shyness, but evolved a sense of relatedness over time. As the interview went on, she became more open about her feelings, and a deepening sense of warmth emerged.

She seemed tense throughout the session. A quality of intensity permeated her speech. There wasn't a lot of variation in her emotion. She alluded to different emotions in the content of her talk, such as being sad when her parents fight and escapist in wanting to run away, or being angry and wanting to hit her brother, but there was little variation in her affect as she talked about these topics. She showed the least flexibility in talking about anger. Her only association was, especially with regard to her parents, to be escapist.

When it came to her thoughts, she showed some capacity to organize her thinking, presenting material in a cohesive manner and adding pieces onto the puzzle after introducing a general theme such as annoyance with her brother. She was able to give some examples of experiences (how she likes to play with her friend at school). In a general sense, then, her thinking seemed organized. However, in particular content areas, she evidenced an inability to maintain a clear distinction between reality and fantasy—the feeling about how cats could talk to her and that creatures from another planet were communicating with her. These experiences were not overwhelming or fragmenting to the rest of her personality. But, at the same time, she was unable to assess these as having a "magical" quality or to debate whether they were real or not. The experiences felt real to her but she also knew they would not be understandable to someone else. They were her "private" communications. For a bright 7-year-old she didn't show an age-appropriate capacity for reality testing (to separate reality from fantasy). In terms of the organization of her thinking, she evidenced a defect.

In a case with this type of difficulty with reality testing, one must always determine the developmental level. What is the nature of the impairment in functioning vis-à-vis age-appropriate expectations? She is able to share attention and engage. She is able to establish two-way gestural communication. She is also able to label some affects and represent certain experiences. For example, she talks about feelings—sad feelings, angry feelings—and elaborates on these (she feels that she wants to beat up her brother). She therefore has some capacity for representational elaboration. In terms of the stages of ego development, she has mastered aspects of attention and engagement, early and more advanced gestural communication, and early representational capacities.

When we come to the next level, the ability for representational differentiation (to form categories and connect experience), she shows a defect in age-appropriate expectations. By age 7, we expect a child not only to have the ability to represent emotional themes and feelings, but to categorize them and make simple connections between these categories. One of the most important categories is reality/fantasy. A 7-year-old should be able to say, "That dream was scary, but it was just a dream." Or, "It feels very real to me, but I know it's just pretend. But it's something that feels so real that I still shut my door and hide under my pillows, because I'm not 100% sure." A 7-year-old may have little islands of belief in magic, "it could happen." "Witches could be real. I don't think they're real, but they could be real."

Seven-year-olds can reason about shades of gray on the fantasy/reality spectrum. Instead, this little girl, when I asked her about the cat, said that there was no question in her mind that the cat talked to her; there was no sense of "well, I think so" or "it sounds unusual." She didn't evidence the ability to separate fantasy and reality and deal with shades of gray.

Consider the sequence of her thinking. She was able to go from one thought to another and make smooth transitions. The sequence of her themes suggested difficulties around anger, particularly her parents' anger and "not talking to each other," and the need to use escapist tendencies. As I later learned, there was much more going on in this family. Subjective reactions included a protective feeling, perhaps a hint of how overwhelmed she was in her family.

In general, she evidenced a significant compromise in age-appropriate capacities in organizing her themes (ideas). She was also below age expectations in her range of themes, range of affects, and her mood. Her capacity to engage and relate, however, was closer to age expectations, as was her ability to remain organized in some aspects of her thematic communication.

CASE 11

Interview

Zachary, a 5½-year-old boy, came in slightly fearful, wanting mother to come with him. He was, however, able to come into the office on his own. There was some caution at first, but gradually he evidenced a nice, warm, engaged quality. He was gentle and a bit clumsy looking, but had good concentration and an even mood. He was slow talking, well connected, slightly hesitant, and shy. He had good understanding of my words and a solid comprehension of the situation. He talked clearly. Occasionally he had a little trouble finding the words he needed to describe something (a bit of a word retrieval or word finding difficulty). For the most part, however, he could find the word if I was patient with him and he took some time with himself.

He first went over to the playhouse, inspecting all the rooms. Then he talked about pictures in the rooms in the playhouse. He described his own house and wanted to know what was outside a door in my office. There was a lot of interest in the office-house being a "big house." He wanted to know if it could be a church.

As he went through the playthings, he found one doll that has many faces on it; one can turn the faces around (a "many-faces" doll). He talked about one "look" being the look of "an evil boy." Another looked "like a witch," and the witch could "cast spells." We discussed the witch casting spells and what the spells could do to people (whether it could cast a spell on all the people or just a few of the people). He never said exactly what he wanted the spell to do, except that it was "magical and powerful."

Then he went to the boy and girl dolls. He showed a great preference for one girl doll with red hair. He said, "I like that doll." He compared it with a boy doll and got into whether he liked the boy or girl doll better, and the advantages of being a boy or a girl. He thought maybe it was better to be a boy "because you can marry a girl." "Boys are stronger, but girls are strong also, but it's bad to want to be a girl, if you're a boy."

As he went on, I could feel the forces working inside him as he was trying to measure the right answers. I empathized with his dilemma, that sometimes it's confusing, and that he has different feelings.

He went back to the many-faces doll and the evil witches hurting "good people." He went from the evil witch hurting the good people to wanting to fix the girl doll with blue hair that was broken a bit. He wanted to use tape to "make it all better." He was careful about taking the tape out and putting it on the arms and legs and trying to attach one leg that was detached. He then had the male hero doll saving the blue girl doll who had been hurt. Then he had the blue girl doll and the red-headed doll biting each other. After a minute, it was not clear whether they were kissing or biting. I tried to clarify what was going on, and he said, "Nothing."

While talking and playing he was holding his genital area in a protective way. (The themes of evil, aggression, people being hurt, injury, self-protection, biting, kissing, and intimacy perhaps are underlying issues that he is struggling with in terms of which gender feels safer and which one is more dangerous.)

Toward the end of the session, he said, "Where's the doctor here?" I said, "What do you mean, where's the doctor?" He said, "Well, I thought I was supposed to see a doctor." He explained that he didn't associate talking and playing with seeing the doctor. He was checking me out and doing a double take. He had a suspicious look, like "What's going on here?" Perhaps he was saying both, "Enough of this stuff," and "When is the real examination going to start?" But at the same time there was a quality of understanding about what was going on. I told him that what we do in here is to talk and play. He compared it with his conception of a doctor as "examining me and giving me shots."

What was interesting here was his perception and the timing of it. After he had gotten fully involved in the session, it was a little late to say, "Hey, who are you, by the way?" I think he had an implicit understanding, but felt at that point maybe he had revealed more than he wanted to, in part about the boy-girl conflicts but also about the underlying feelings about good and evil and aggression. Yet, he remained organized, verbal, and in an even mood for the entire session. Near the end of the session, I asked him to draw some pictures and he showed reasonably good fine motor control.

I was impressed in his first session that his basic personality functions, of reality testing, relatedness, concentration, impulse control, and stable mood, were intact and age-appropriate. He was slightly cautious and there was a question of secrets. He was trying to say what he thought was right to say, but he also clearly revealed that there were lots of issues around good-evil and aggression, and how to protect himself. These were connected in his mind with the boy-girl conflicts.

In the next session, he again came in very engaged, looking a little bit confused, with a joyful, relaxed quality. He evidenced a sophisticated use of language, good attention, and an even mood. His themes focused on looking in the castle, opening and closing things, the castle being scary, and wanting to know what was in every corner and nook. This was similar to the first theme of the first session when we were exploring the house, and looking behind closed doors (exploring the mysteries of life). This interest may be associated with feelings about his own body (the sense of mystery of it), and/or his fantasies about his parents who had evidenced considerable conflict during his early childhood and were now separated.

The castle suddenly became scary. He said it was a "haunted castle." He got two castles down and made up quite an elaborate drama. The figures were going up this or that stairway, getting stuck, etc. He was very clever in the way he created a fantasy around the spatial qualities of the castles.

He was richer in his fantasy creations this time than in the first session. He was also more engaged and warmer. He then compared the castles with "Dad's house" and "Mom's house." The theme of mystery emerged again. Then he picked up the boy and girl dolls and said, "Better to be a daddy because I am a boy." He related the boy and girl to the different houses. "But Mom's house is better because it is more beautiful." He was intrigued with things that are "beautiful." He subsequently said, "To be a girl is more fun, because you can wear dresses, and you can be beautiful."

He then mentioned his parents' separation and his view that they lived apart because they "fought a lot, and they're not married anymore." He talked about being "strong like a man" versus "being beautiful," and the pros and cons of both.

In a third session, he again started out cautious, wanting father to come in with him. He came in on his own, however, and was silent for a few minutes. He then got right into play themes. He found a doll's dress in the toy closet and wanted to know where the girl was. He thought maybe the dress had come off one of the girl dolls. He got right into the theme of girl versus boy, in terms of dresses versus pants, and the different hair on different dolls. He wondered which one was nice and not nice, and which color he liked and didn't like, etc. Then he elaborated on how their bodies were different. When I inquired about these differences, he talked about the "penis" versus the "vagina" as another difference. He thought it was "better to have a vagina. A peepee looks funny because the peepee comes out from the bottom. It looks funny, and the vagina doesn't stick out."

Then he said, "Penises can hurt sometimes." He talked about taking a bath and about the penis being small versus big. Themes of hurting again were mentioned. (I think he was talking about erections, and how it's big when he plays with it or takes a bath, and either it hurts him or he feels it is vulnerable to being hurt.) The themes continued to have something that sticks out, something that hurts or can be hurt, and something that can get small and big.

His next associations were of good and bad people and princesses, and a video game–type savior who could help people when they were in danger. The theme of danger was eminent, and there were battles between good and bad. As he was elaborating, he ignored me when I asked questions, intermittently tuning me out.

Subsequently, he talked about wanting to dress up as a girl, and how one of the girl dolls was beautiful. Then he said, "My mom is beautiful." There was a clear association between his own desire to be beautiful, the doll being beautiful, and his mom being beautiful.

He also said that if he had his choice he would rather be a beautiful girl than a powerful boy; that he knew he should be a boy, but that in his heart he was interested more in being beautiful and a girl.

Comments

As indicated, Zachary's capacities to relate, interact, and represent experience were all age-appropriate. His mood, affects, and themes were all stable and organized. He also evidenced marked constrictions in the age-expected range of affects and themes. He focused on core conflicts to the exclusion of age-appropriate themes. Instead of pleasure in assertiveness, pride in his body, and confidence in expanding peer relationships and interests, his associations were of themes of danger, worrying about his penis being hurt, dramas of good versus evil, being saved by a powerful video game–type person, and being beautiful and being like his mother, and therefore preferring to be a girl. These themes were expressed more at the level of representational elaboration than representational differentiation. The idealizations, denials, and fears were not connected other than by association. While he had some capacities to create bridges between his representations, there were also undifferentiated islands related to his areas of conflict and constriction. My subjective reaction was to feel protective in terms of challenging or exploring too rapidly his concerns, suggesting perhaps a sense of underlying fragility.

In general, therefore, he evidenced capacities below age expectations in the areas of affective range, thematic range, and thematic organization. His relationship capacity, mood, and ability to concentrate were closer to age expectations.

CASE 12

Interview

For a few moments, I was able to observe Mark in the waiting room with his parents. He was a blond-haired 4½-year-old, extremely tall, strongly and thickly built. He walked with an unusual gait, stepping first onto his toes, then flopping down to his heels, while his arms moved every which way in a purposeless but not quite spastic fashion. I saw him toss a ball to his father and follow instructions from his parents. When I offered my hand to him and asked him to come into the office, he refused and moved away from me in his special, uncoordinated style, running to his mother's lap. After a few moments of patient, expectant waiting, I suggested that the family come in together.

In the playroom Mark seemed able to understand and carry out even complex instructions from his parents, which they eagerly volunteered. ("Show Dr. Greenspan how you play.") The child quickly made eye contact with me and even started to move in my direction, but then made a fast retreat and jumped in mother's lap. His father insisted that he get down and play, which he did. His quality of relatedness to me, and even somewhat to his parents, was unusual in that he would make fleeting contact and then seemingly lose contact, his eyes taking on a glazed, preoccupied appearance. Unlike a youngster who makes contact and then becomes negative and breaks it off, Mark would make a quick contact and then seem to become confused or disorganized. After such contact he would shift in another direction and often behave aimlessly for a few moments.

During the early part of the interview, while his parents were encouraging him to play, he would say things—e.g., "The wolf is coming"—from out of the blue. When he commented that the wolf was coming, he was not playing with the toy wolf, nor had there been any prior mention of animals or of people being attacked. On occasion throughout the interview he would start to approach me, then change this action to running to mother or father and wanting to be held. At times, he would aggressively pinch mother or father, and they would become angry and slap him, insisting that he "go back on the floor and show Dr. Greenspan how you play."

In about the middle of the interview Mark got angry, seemingly without provocation, and started screaming, "I want to go." This outburst rapidly took on the quality of a tantrum as he stamped up and down and jumped about with his floppy leg movements and uncoordinated arm movements. His voice had a slightly gruff quality but was clear and distinct. His statement, "I want to go," was the most purposeful one he made during the entire interview. When his parents did not respond to this demand, he went over and pinched one of them. Then he proceeded to wander around the room for a few minutes in a seemingly confused state. He did not approach any of the toys or other play materials; he did not develop any activity.

After he had explored a little of the room in this random way, he went to mother and somewhat gently sat in her lap and cuddled in her arms. Within a moment of seeming to be warm to her, he said, "I hurt you if we don't go." Mother responded supportively, again directing him to the toys on the floor. He was then able to begin building a tower of blocks. This was by far his most organized performance during the session. While their son was thus engaged in focused concentration, father appeared to be uncomfortable and mother seemed to show sympathy and warmth. At one point father insisted, "Get me a duck from over there." This command had the effect of distracting Mark's focus on building the tower.

As the interview progressed, mother looked increasingly depressed and withdrawn; she did not seem to know how to "get Mark to perform better." Father grew increasingly impatient, and his sporadic outbursts of "do this" and "do that" became angry demands. Meanwhile, Mark continued to explore the toys in his random way. He touched things and occasionally put little dolls or blocks in his mouth. At one point his mother asked him what color something was and he was able to say it was orange; then his father asked him to spell it and he spelled it correctly.

At times Mark would refuse to get down from his mother's lap by saying, "I want to sit on your lap." Once when he was sitting there, he put a pencil in his mouth and began holding his genitals. Sometimes when he walked around, he would begin almost shaking with excitement, stretching out his arms in every direction and moving his fingers and arms up and down randomly. He occasionally said words that were incomprehensible, seemingly tying together syllables from different words. He also uttered sentences from out of the blue, such as, "I have poison in my mouth." At one point, when his parents did not do what he asked, he threatened to stab them with a pencil and excitedly went at them until his father grabbed him. Throughout most of the interview his affects were bland and flat, although he showed chaotic excitement or confused bewilderment from time to time, as well as exhibiting an occasional interest in being held.

Near the end of the interview, still trying to demonstrate Mark's abilities, father asked him to name things, and he was able to identify many objects in the room. Father also got a book to show me how Mark could identify the pictures—which Mark did very well. Indeed, he demonstrated an overall ability to identify objects at or above his chronological age. Father also asked him to spell a few additional words, which he was able to do.

This pattern of showing occasional interest in the play material, wandering around the room, and jumping into mother's lap continued till the end of the interview, when Mark seemed happy to be able to leave with his parents. He showed little relatedness in saying good-bye; he looked away from me as he was leaving the office.

Comments

This 4½-year-old boy showed some worrisome features in his overall physical and neurological development, that is, his unusual gait and uncoordinated arm movements. In many respects, his gait was reminiscent of a 14- or 15-month-old not yet comfortable with walking. He was able to understand and formulate words reasonably well, however, and in play with some objects his fine motor coordination looked fairly good. His language and aspects of cognitive functioning with structure appeared more advanced than his general ability to communicate. His activity level was highly uneven—occasionally relaxed and focused, but often excited and very reactive. His overall mood seemed to be one of confusion and disorganization, with occasional breakthroughs of frustrated feelings and rage. His affect was mostly bland and flat except for occasional shifts to an undifferentiated excited state or to a mild, partly frustrated, angry state. The absence of subtlety or range in his affect placed him well below age expectations in this category.

As described above, Mark made fleeting eye contact with me. He made more contact with his parents, especially his mother; he wanted to sit in her lap and be cuddled. To me, his relatedness seemed disorganized, reminiscent of an 8- to 15-month-old having stranger anxiety. There was a worried look on his face when he glanced at me. For the most part, however, he did not relate to anyone other than mother, thus indicating that his capacity for relatedness was well below age expectations.

He seemed chronically anxious during the interview. The few themes that emerged concerned wolves, attacks, or poison. I speculated that his anxiety may have been related to fear of annihilation and bodily damage as well as to the more obvious concern about separation from mother. He was highly disorganized in his capacities to communicate with me and to develop any coherent themes. Most dramatic was the fragmented, piecemeal quality of his communications. On the whole, his behavior seemed random and chaotic, far below age expectations for a 4½-year-old. His gestural and presymbolic behavioral communications lacked intentionality and organization. (These capacities are ordinarily established in the second year of life.) While partially engaged, he lacked full mastery of focused attention, two-way gestural communication, and representational capacities.

The fragmented themes that emerged were wishing to be close to mother, feelings of violence when frustrated (e.g., "I'll stick a pencil in you"), and concerns about wolves attacking and being poisoned. There was general apprehension about exploring, interspersed with climbing into mother's lap for what appeared to be security and safety. Thus, the sequence of themes suggested concerns about separation and the most fundamental issues of security, anger, and safety. In addition, a pronounced inability to deal with frustrated, angry impulses was evidenced by the overall disorganized quality of his communications.

My subjective reactions were concern for the explosive, violent quality that occasionally emerged, and exhaustion from watching the parents try to help their child become more organized, as well as father's overdemanding intrusive approach. My initial impression was that this child was significantly below age expectations in most areas of functioning, including important areas such as relating to others and organizing communications. One exception was his well-developed capacity to name objects and spell, suggesting that aspects of intellectual functioning may be at age level.

CASE 13

First Interview

Molly, a 4½-year-old, readily turned to me when I entered the waiting room. Showing a trace of eagerness on her otherwise expressionless face, she followed me into the office. She was well-built, slightly stocky, of average height, and walked in a clearly coordinated though somewhat "unfeminine" manner. Later in the interview she showed, through manipulation of crayons and drawing pencils, that her fine motor coordination was also quite well developed.

When she came into the room she gave me a rather straightforward yet cold look and asked in a slightly domineering tone, "Do you have a lollipop?" When I did not respond immediately, she explained, "I didn't get breakfast today. I threw up, I was sick." I commented that she must feel very hungry, and in return she gave me an expressionless look. Then she began to walk around and explore the room, occasionally turning toward me and commenting about what she saw, naming an ashtray and a book. Her vocabulary, her capacity for naming things, and her overall perceptiveness seemed quite well developed. As she talked and made eye contact with me, however, there was no expression of joy or pleasure. At times a sad, even depressed, quality came through.

After a brief exploration, she went to one corner of the room where she stood rather rigidly for the rest of the session. I went to where she was standing and apparently looking at a few objects on the table. She asked if I would be interested to "see how I can take off my shirt," adding quickly, "but I don't want to." Again there was a sad look; no flirtatious or joyous affect was associated with this comment. As a matter of fact, the discontinuity between her verbalization and her emotionless expression was striking.

After a few more minutes of looking around, she volunteered, "I like stuffed animals." She then named a few things in the room and said, "I want to take these home." At one point she said she wanted to take the soap from the bathroom home. Such comments were often isolated and followed by silences. She did not say, for example, "Gee, there are many things here I would like to take home," and then list the items. A quality of affect hunger began to emerge and I could feel empathic concern for her. However, because the emotional expression was so blank, my empathic reaction was not as strong as one might expect in such circumstances.

The theme of wanting to take things home dominated the remainder of the interview. She would play with a toy silently, look at me, and say, "I want this one." She then put all her selections in a corner of the room. She left the room without trying to take the toys, much as she had come, in a striding gait and with little emotional expression.

Comments on First Interview

My impression was that Molly was a physically and neurologically intact 4½-year-old, as evidenced by her gross and fine motor coordination, use of language, and overall healthy appearance. There was a capacity for relating but it had little variation, richness, or depth and developed only to the point of expressions of affect hunger. She showed little warmth or intimacy, nor was she demanding or interested in a power struggle. Molly's capacity for relatedness seemed to be at a very concrete, early developmental level; she related like a somewhat sad and needy 2- to 3-year-old.

The mood, as already described, seemed mostly depressed and constricted. The range of affect was quite narrow. Little was expressed beyond a mildly constricted or flattened quality and a degree of affect hunger around the themes of wanting to take things home. There was no affective demonstration of joy, curiosity, seductiveness, compassion, or empathy, nor were there signs of rage, protest, jealousy, or envy. In short, none of the age-appropriate affects were to be seen. The affects that were visible were well below age expectations—again, more like those of a constricted 2-year-old.

Molly showed a capacity to organize her themes. There were no overt fragmentations, no comments or themes from out of the blue. But there was little depth or richness to her thematic development; in other words, it was shallow and concrete. Her shallow and impoverished thematic patterns were limited to asking if I had a lollipop, naming things in the room, standing in a corner and wanting to take off her shirt, and telling me the kinds of toys she liked and all the things she wanted to take home.

Developmentally, there was a capacity to engage, to communicate intentionally with gestures, and to elaborate and differentiate representations, but with severe constrictions at every level.

The thematic sequence progressed from wanting something from me to an interest in exploring the room; the latter was followed first by inhibition, as she lodged herself in one quarter of the room, and then by a desire to show herself, which was quickly contradicted; finally she showed a desire for me to get to know her likes and dislikes of various toys (which also had the sense that she was telling me what she might like from me as a present). None of these themes was developed. Finally, near the end of the interview, she was telling me clearly that she wanted to take things home, and her statements were accompanied by a sense of affect hunger. The sequence suggests a little girl who feels quite hungry at a concrete level, who has concretized some of her human needs, and who is too frightened to let people know her. Although she wants to get close (by taking off her shirt), to reveal some of her needs, and to move into exhibitionistic themes, there is no accompanying affect and she becomes inhibited and returns to the theme of making concrete demands of the interviewer. One might hypothesize that strong conflicts are inhibiting a greater development in the sequence; perhaps conflicts around early primitive rage that accompanies some of this concretization, and around affect hunger. Because many questions remained after the first diagnostic interview, a second interview was conducted.

Second Interview

In the second interview, Molly entered the playroom much as she had done in the first, demonstrating good gross and fine motor ability and a clear capacity for vocalization. She was not expressionless, however; there was an intense, depressed look on her face. Moreover, her eye contact was engaging rather than aloof. She also showed less initial tentativeness and demonstrated a capacity to communicate in a clear and organized way. After moving around to survey the room in a slightly more relaxed fashion than she had previously shown, Molly sat down on the beanbag, looked at me (although still maintaining the intense, depressed look on her face), and said, "If you think of scary things sometimes, you won't breathe." She then continued to talk almost nonstop for the remainder of the session while she sat on the beanbag or walked around. For the most part she kept eye contact with me in an intense, somewhat depressed look, but showed some emotional variation—a smile here, a look of bewilderment there.

At first she talked about robbers and killers hurting other people and herself, and then she stood up and pretended that she was a "rocket ship" that was going to "take off." She then came back to the theme of robbers and killers. When I asked her to say more about it, she replied that they could kill you by cutting you with a "knife," that they could take your "eyes out," that they could "break off in your stomach."

Then she made a reference to her younger brother. When I asked her about him, she quickly changed the subject and said, "At school no one likes me—they hate me." There followed a brief silence; then she said, "kill them." When I picked up on this phrase, her serious and intense look shifted to a mild smirk and she said, "but only pretend." She talked more about killing and being killed. After I made a summary comment, she said, "Family—they don't want me to die, they like me." She made a confused reference to not breathing again, but would not elaborate on it.

A few minutes later, while walking around and exploring the room, she commented, "I like my shape. I'm a girl. It's different from my brother because I have long hair." I offered a summary comment to encourage her to talk more about how she differed from her brother, but Molly only repeated what she had said and then spontaneously drew a "snake": a long oval shape with two legs sticking out the back, two arms sticking out the middle, and the face of a little girl (the sex was evidenced by the long hair around the face). As I took an interest in the drawing and began wondering aloud about it, she said something about it being "a snake that can't see females"; then her words became confused, but I heard, "it's poison." She scribbled around the image, then drew pictures of two or three more snakes and said spontaneously, "That's me. . . . If I look at it, I can't breathe." She abruptly put the drawings aside and, with a rather serious but inanimate look on her face, went to the other side of the room where she started naming objects.

As in the first interview, she wanted to know if there were things she could take home, such as a checkers set, some crayons, and paper cups and soap from the bathroom. I commented that she was telling me it was scary to look at a poisonous snake and that perhaps taking some things with her from the office would make her feel less afraid. Looking at me as though to take in the supplied connection, she simply reiterated her wish to have these things. While her affect as well as the sense of relatedness remained tense and depressed throughout, there was no disorganization or fragmentation to her themes. When the interview ended, she looked at me to say good-bye, and the expression on her face seemed to indicate a desire to return.

Comments on Second Interview

During Molly's second interview, I again saw that neurological and physical functioning were at the age-appropriate level. With regard to her sense of relatedness, although she was a little more involved and somewhat more intimate than she had been during the first interview, she was still highly constricted. There was also constriction in the sense of rigidity and distance she created—despite the fact that she communicated a great deal. As before, her mood was tense and depressed, although she showed slightly more variation. Although her affect was again very constricted, there was a greater range than in the first interview. There were momentary smirks and smiles, and a few instances of something near to curiosity and pleasure in what she was doing. Her affect was not as flat; she showed a tense, more rigid quality this time, a sense of seriousness. The affect was also slightly richer and deeper than during the first interview.

Molly showed some anxiety during the second interview, particularly after drawing the snakes, when she went to the other side of room and talked about the concrete objects she wanted to take home. There was no disorganization as a result of her anxiety, but neither was there a capacity to use anxiety as a signal and then return to its source, i.e., the drawings. Instead, she avoided the anxiety by almost pretending that the drawings were not there. There was some indication that the anxiety had to do with the themes of being poisoned or hurt.

Thematic organization was more in evidence during this interview than in the first. She showed a capacity to organize a number of themes—especially while drawing the snakes—and to integrate her communication around one specific theme that was obviously troubling her. There was greater depth and richness to the themes during this interview than during the first one: themes of hurting, cutting, taking eyes out, not being liked, hating, and being different from her brother, as well as feelings about poisonous, aggressive snakes. This thematic development was in only one or two dimensions, however—that of aggression and hatred and their consequences, and hints of concerns with being a girl versus a boy (her brother). There was little thematic development in the other sectors that one would expect to see in a 4½-year-old.

Developmentally, we see here, as in the first interview, a capacity for engagement and two-way gestural communication, and representational elaboration and differentiation. In this interview, one is impressed with the intensity of her representational concerns, the suggested conflicts, and the areas of emotion that are not represented.

The thematic sequence revealed the nature of her drama. It progressed from fears of not breathing, to robbers and killers, to herself taking off like an explosive rocket ship, to eyes being cut out with knives, to others not liking her in school, to her family not wanting her to die, to being a girl and being interested in her own shape, to the poisonous snake who she says is herself, and then to a quick shift to her hunger to take concrete things home. All of these themes pointed to her preoccupation with aggression, bodily injuries, and death.

There was some indication that her emerging sexual identity was somewhat tied up in this frightening imagery, making it hard for her to feel comfortable about being a little girl. When she was too close to seeing herself as an aggressive, poisonous snake, she needed to switch to a more concrete mode and express her wish to take things home with her. Thus, at the point of anxiety when she came closest to her frightening self-image, she sought reassurances via a regressive, concrete tie to another person. Such a move suggests some fear of object loss. This fear seemed to be tremendous and close to the surface, actuated continuously by the aggressive themes. The pattern seems to be: she experiences a need; she feels "poisonous" and becomes fearful of loss; she then wants concrete objects as reassurances.

In this interview we see a number of age-appropriate areas of functioning (e.g., physical-neurological, thematic organization, affect organization). But we also observe below-age-appropriate functioning to a significant degree in her constrictions of affective and thematic range and depth, her style of relatedness, and her special thematic preoccupations.

INTERVIEWS WITH INFANTS, VERY YOUNG CHILDREN, AND THEIR PARENTS

The following interviews were with children under age 4 years. With very young children, the clinical interview will involve the interaction of parent(s) and the child. The clinician, after observing, may join in and interact with the child or the child and the parent(s). The same observational framework that we applied to older children may also be used for younger children. With younger children, however, we naturally focus on the earlier developmental/organizational processes and the early aspects of each aspect of development (relationships, affects, etc.). It should be pointed out that just as with older children, clinical work with infants and very young children requires special training and experience. For a detailed description of the clinical assessment and treatment of infants, young children, and their families, see *Emotional and Developmental Disorders of Infancy and Early Childhood: Clinical Assessment and Treatment* (Greenspan 1991).

CASE 14

Interview

Eddie, 3½ years old, was sitting next to his mother in the waiting room. I was impressed by his large face, glasses, and strong, scholarly look. He came and stood very close to me when I entered the waiting room, and I noticed that he walked in a comfortable, almost adamant manner with a slightly broadened gait. He quickly showed that his fine motor coordination was good by the way he held a pencil and made shapes while drawing freely. Spontaneously, he took the drawings he had made from his mother and handed them to me as though he were doing it on her behalf. His voice initially had a slightly nasal, monotonous quality as he spoke in response to my introducing myself and asking his name.

He came into the office on his own, leaving mother in the

waiting room, and immediately sat down and started scribbling on a piece of paper. He mentioned the words "mommy" and "daddy" and again told me his name. His drawing was mostly scribbles and lines; I asked what it was and he said, "Big body, big boy." He then found a doll, said, "I got dolly," and proceeded to point out and name the ears, arms, feet ("eats"), and mouth. He then started twisting the doll's arm and grimacing, as though he could understand it was hurting. "Ouch,"he said. I commented empathically that it must hurt. He responded, "I like you. Hurt if I like, I like to, I like to." When I picked up on his use of the word "like," repeating things he likes, he said, "Throw him up, not hurt. Throw up high," and made reference to the doll's hands and mouth. He then grabbed a toy dog and again said, "Throw up. Play with doggy." He was playing in a less aggressive way with the toy dog and I commented, "You seem to enjoy playing with the doggy." He responded "Yes," and hiccupped. He then stood up, almost wobbling, and played while standing.

At this point he seemed pensive. I commented that it seemed he had a picture of something in his mind. He said, "Mommy. Like to get Mommy for Daddy for office because like to." He then made a reference to needing money and wanting to count pennies. Then he came and stood almost on top of me, showing little facial expression and not looking in my direction. For a moment he stood still, but then he began shaking the toy dog and hitting its head. He gave a big yawn, then proceeded to say phrases: "I like to," "I got to you," "Mommy, doggy, and fun." He seemed to be moving even closer to me and to be getting uncomfortable, as though he wanted to relate but could not. He gave me a blank stare. I commented that he seemed to want to tell me something. He said, "Red point in mind."

There was very little variation in emotional tone or affect during this time. He was obviously struggling with something, judging by the very serious look on his face. He began pulling on his fingers and said, "Getting yack off because I like to." He put his fingers in his mouth and wandered around the room, looking at me blankly. I commented that maybe he did not know what to do and suggested that perhaps he could tell me a little about Mommy and Daddy. He said, "Daddy and Mommy come here and I stay with babysitters . . . I like babysitters." When I asked him to tell me more about this, he became visibly anxious, put his hands on his neck, and said, "Mommy likes babysitters, that's all." He then went over to touch some of the toys but was tentative and seemed almost afraid to touch them. He referred to a duck and to Big Bird on TV, commented that he had toys at home, and again positioned himself very near but not quite touching me.

Near the end of the interview I asked if he ever had dreams (describing what I meant), and he responded with, "Hurting, headache, go out." I asked him if his head hurt when he slept. He pointed to his head and repeated the word "headache" while standing very close to me in a rigid posture, with a kind of adamant, serious, joyless look on his face. When I ended the interview, he went out to the waiting room without much facial expression or attention to me, and he returned to his mother in a similar way.

Comments

Although there were some questions about Eddie's gait, his gross and fine motor and sensory processing capacities were age-appropriate. His comprehension of my questions, while inconsistent, reflected an ability to comprehend some verbal statements. He articulated his words and sentences clearly. His mood had a general, almost unvaried, apprehensive quality. In terms of relatedness, an underlying intense hunger was expressed through physical closeness, but little actual emotional warmth was manifested. Eddie's relatedness had a hungry yet impersonal quality. There was little range of affect. His affects seemed contained and constrained; there was little show of joy or pleasure, and no actual outbursts of anger or protest accompanying the various thematic developments. Anxiety seemed to be generalized. On the whole, the interview had a fragmented quality to it.

Thematic organization, in terms of representational capacity, was not age-appropriate for a 3½-year-old in that there was no development of organized themes through play material or verbal expression. We saw a lot of pieces of representational communication in the context of some relatedness. There was little depth or richness to the themes. Most 3½-year-olds are able to communicate at an interactive and play level by integrating some verbalization with their play actions, as well as being logical in their discussions. He could be differentiated only part of the time.

Developmentally, he was intentional in his use of gestures, but was quite fragmented in his representational capacities. He did comprehend the structure of the playroom.

The thematic sequence proceeded as follows. We saw an initial interest in the body parts of a doll and in hurting the doll ("Ouch"); indications of liking the interviewer; and concerns with not hurting, with throwing things up, with wanting to "like" the toy dog or be close to it, with thinking about parents and "liking" or being "close to" Mommy, and with needing money. The themes evolved from concerns about body parts and hurtfulness, to ambivalence about hurting and liking (with liking being more related to Mommy, and hurting more related to Daddy), to concerns with accumulating money, to fun and hurting again (hitting the dog's head). The theme of moving close to and then away from me, suggesting ambivalence about accumulating or wanting things, followed. My attempt to help him express what was on his mind evoked the theme of the "red point," pulling things off his fingers, and putting fingers in his mouth. When asked about parents, he indicated that perhaps he gets the babysitters instead of his parents. When asked to talk about mother, he put his hands around his neck, again indicating some tension and anxiety, and said only, "Mommy likes babysitters." He related dreams to hurting and headaches. This thematic sequence, although disjointed, and more in the pattern of a 2½-year-old (i.e., representational elaboration without much representational differentiation), gives us some clues to his concerns and possible conflicts.

Notice that no single theme was developed to any depth. Being close to Mommy had something to do with choking or strangulation in an aggressive yet unrelated sense, perhaps indicating that more time was spent with the babysitter than with mother. After the choking theme, Eddie returned to an impersonal desire to accumulate (tentatively touching toys) as a way of handling the need for dependency. His response to dreams demonstrated additional concern with aggression and physical pain. In sum, we saw a child excessively concerned with aggression and injury and with very little warmth, whose overall thematic capacity for organization, depth, and richness was well below age expectations.

Concerning the organization of affect around themes, Eddie seemed preoccupied with issues of ambivalence. He was ambivalent about being close to people, and both ambivalent and angry about hurting people. He hinted that he suffered "headaches" as a result of these conflicts. Overall, he was below age-appropriate functioning in terms of thematic affect organization, although he showed some depth in this respect.

In summary, there was some capacity for relatedness and for separation from mother. In the former, he was highly constricted, however, showing little warmth or sense of personal relatedness. Mood stability was slightly below age expectations. Other major functions, notably thematic organization and depth and richness of affect, were significantly below age expectations. In these areas he was functioning at about the 2- to 3-year-old level. On the basis of this interview material, therefore, one would be concerned about uneven personality development in this child. As with all the cases presented in this book, a complete workup including further interviews, careful family evaluations, detailed developmental history, and appropriate developmental studies as needed is required to follow up on the impressions from any one interview.

CASE 15

Interview

Jane was cute and well built, although somewhat small for her age of 2 years, 11 months. As I entered the waiting room, she was standing, holding her mother's knee. She looked over in my direction and presented a kind of prepared look, as though she knew why she was there. Mother, after greeting me, quickly got together some toys that she had brought in a bag. (I had asked her to bring some of Jane's favorite toys.) They came into the office with me and sat down on the floor. As Jane walked into the room, she showed basically good gross motor coordination and gait. Mother took out some toys and suggested that Jane play with them. Jane looked over in my direction and around the room a bit with a solemn yet interested and curious expression. Although her facial expression was not animated, she projected some apprehension and tension. Mother also seemed slightly anxious, but promptly got down to business, offering the child a car and Lego blocks. Jane quickly began putting together some of the Legos, demonstrating excellent dexterity with her fingers and fine motor coordination.

As Jane began playing with the Legos, her mother began a running commentary, describing the child's activities. She looked directly at Jane as she spoke but also seemed to be doing it for my benefit. For instance, when Jane started rolling a toy car back and forth, mother said, "Oh, now you are playing with a car." Jane also talked as she played, saying, "I want the doll, give me the truck," etc. She was able to give a commentary of sorts as to what she was doing and to identify toys as she took them out—"That's a Lego, that's a cow," etc.

During this time Jane was clearly relating at an emotional level to both her mother and me, looking at mother and occasionally glancing in my direction. When she glanced at me, I smiled, and when I thought she was saying to me, "That's a cow," I commented, "Yes, it is," to make myself available for involvement in the play. However, it was also noticeable that there was little change in Jane's facial expression; while very involved in manipulating the toys and verbalizing what she was doing (I should mention her verbal capacity was at the level of short sentences), Jane showed little range of affect or emotion. Instead, there was a constant apprehensive look to her face. There were, for example, no occasions when she broke into bright, excited, or gleeful smiles; nor were there any occasions when she became negativistic, stubborn, or seemingly angry.

Also noticeable was that Jane and her mother sat almost entirely in one spot. Jane moved to take things from the bag of toys but not to explore the room. She specifically did not show any interest in the toys that were in my toy closet, which was well within her eyesight. Finally, about 20 minutes into the interview, she looked over at my toys, and mother suggested that she might like to see what "Dr. Greenspan's toys were like." With that bit of encouragement, Jane got up and walked to the toy closet. She took out a block and said, "This is a block. I will build a house." Mother then helped her take out a number of blocks and Jane began piling them up. At this point she was showing a little greater interest and curiosity and some slight relaxation, although the affect still remained mildly apprehensive.

Again, in piling up the blocks, Jane showed a good capacity to concentrate and to focus on what she was doing. She took out toy cars and a truck, naming them as she did so. She then took out a gun, looked perplexed, and said, "What is this?" Mother said, "That's a gun," and then explained, "We don't have them at home." Except for helping each other with the materials, there was little direct interaction between mother and Jane around any of the play activities.

Soon Jane found a hand puppet in the form of a fish. She put it on her hand and said, "This is a fish. It's going to bite you, Mommy," then thrust it toward mother's face. Mother quickly drew back and, quickly and very aggressively taking the puppet away and onto her own hand, said, "It's going to bite *you*." Then Jane took it back from her, and mother, with a somewhat reflex response, extended her finger and let Jane pretend to bite it with the fish puppet. Subsequently Jane took out a duck puppet and played the same game. This time mother extended her finger in a more relaxed fashion. Again, mother withdrew rather abruptly when Jane went after her face. Although she did not take it away from Jane, she said, "The duck is going to bite *you*."

Mother seemed interested in evolving some interactive play with Jane around this theme of the fish or duck biting her, but only to a slight degree. She did not take advantage of this interactive sequence to build on it by developing any associations or story line. For example, she did not say, "What is the duck going to do next?" or "The duck has strong feelings" or "The duck likes to bite." There was also a mildly apprehensive look on mother's face during this more aggressive play. Jane put down the duck on her own after playing with it for a few minutes and then returned to removing items from the toy cabinet and naming them. She did this with a fairly comfortable, curious quality, although again she showed little joy or pleasure.

Shortly thereafter, Jane went back to sit on the floor with her own toys. Mother suggested that she show me her newest game, which was a small magnetized chalkboard with letters that attached to it. Jane took out the chalk and showed me that she could draw some lines. I then sat down on the floor and made myself available to her on a more physically intimate level. Jane initially responded to this by standing up behind her mother as though mildly apprehensive. After a minute or two of this she was able to come back and sit down next to me and show me how she could take the chalk and draw a line. I then drew a circle and asked her if she could copy that. She was able to do a fairly decent circle with only one side of it drawn more like a square. I then drew an X and she copied it, but drew just a single line. Mother suggested that she show me the letters, and Jane found the letter A, saying, "Abbey."

Mother, for the first time showing a truly joyful smile, said, "I didn't know you could do that." Mother explained to me that Abbey was Jane's sister's name. Jane then went on to name other letters, being able to do so on her own about 70% of the time with mother helping her about 30% of the time. Mother seemed proud, but indicated she had worked with Jane on this and was well aware that she could name these letters. What surprised her was that Jane could find the letter that matched the sister's name. As Jane was naming the letters, I too demonstrated pride and said things like, "That's terrific." Jane looked up at me, acknowledging the compliment, and then busily went back to name some more. Here again, however, she showed few signs of overt pleasure but instead maintained her chronic apprehensiveness.

During this phase of the activity with mother, Jane, and me sitting together, the interaction was probably as comfortable as possible. In other words, even though Jane was mildly apprehensive and mother was busy encouraging her to name the letters, there was some sense of underlying relaxation. Subjectively, I felt that Jane was then probably as relaxed with me as she gets with most people, even though she had been with me only about 40 minutes at that point.

The interview continued in this vein until I suggested that we would have to stop in a minute. Jane took in those directions, and she helped mother put the letters and toys back in their places. During this time Jane was able to make good eye contact with me, accompanying her apprehensive look with a smile. After putting the toys away, mother got Jane's coat on and they prepared to leave. Jane was able to look at me and say good-bye as mother and I arranged another appointment before they left.

Comments

Jane demonstrated that her overall physical and neurological status was within age-appropriate guidelines. Although on the small side, she was physically well built and well proportioned. She had good gross and fine motor coordination, could understand and formulate words clearly and talk in sentences, and showed an excellent capacity to name items and letters. Her capacity to name the letters was probably a bit above age expectations, as was the capacity to match the appropriate letter with her sister's first name.

With respect to her relatedness, there was clearly a capacity for human relatedness, as demonstrated in the waiting room when she had her hand on mother's leg. For an almost 3-year-old, perhaps this showed a desire to be especially close to mother and to forgo the curiosity and explorative activities one might expect. She also clearly showed a capacity to relate to me by making immediate eye contact and acknowledging my presence even when she was playing with mother on the floor and I was sitting in my chair. This capacity was also demonstrated by her frequent glances at me and by including both mother and me when she was talking or naming things, even though it was also clear that the relatedness to me was more indirect.

Once I sat down and joined them on the floor, there was a sense of three people relating to one another and Jane was able to interact with me, follow my instructions, and look at me. There was a sense of warmth that came through in spite of the apprehensiveness. This quality of warmth should not be underestimated, as it demonstrated that her capacity for human relatedness was well founded. I would speculate, however—more by way of inference than by observation—that there is some restriction in the range of affect in her relatedness as well as in her sense of exploration, the latter evidenced especially by the extent to which she stayed close to mother during most of the time in the playroom.

Her mood, as reported, had an apprehensive and slightly anxious quality throughout the session. Even at the end, when warmth and relaxation came through a bit, there was no general sense of relaxation. There was very little variation in the mood, which overall seemed stable.

Constriction seemed to be present in the range of affects. There was the mild apprehension, only a slight show of curiosity and interest, and little genuinely gleeful happiness. Although there were some mild signs of aggressiveness, there was no accompanying affect. For example, when Jane tried to bite her mother's nose and finger with the hand puppets, she always did so with the same apprehensive and nervous look on her face rather than with a gleeful playfulness, an out-of-control belligerence, or a hostile negativism. In fact, none of these affect ranges were present during the interview. At no time was the affect inappropriate to the theme she was developing, however, and there was an overall sense of connectedness and warmth, as reported above. Her persistently apprehensive affect was not shallow in terms of connectedness and warmth.

There were no abrupt shifts or disorganizations during the interview stemming from anxiety. Generally, she maintained her focus on each play theme until she seemed to want to shift. That anxiety might have been present was indicated by her chronically apprehensive, nervous quality and by her need to stay physically closer to mother than one might expect of a child her age—perhaps indicative of an underlying separation anxiety. There were also some indications that mother had difficulty handling Jane's aggression, as when mother quickly turned the table with the hand puppets, saying, "It's going to bite *you*." Perhaps such a response signifies mother's underlying fear of being attacked. Again, the above comments are speculations based more on inference than on direct observations.

Jane seemed capable of developing organized themes in little islands of play; for example, when she took out the toys, there was the theme of naming things and exploration. Then there were the themes of building the house and showing how she could name letters. Within each "thematic island" she was focused, organized, and cohesive, but she lacked the age-appropriate capacity for developing depth or richness. One would expect a 2½- to 3-year-old as bright and organized as Jane to develop a bit further themes like "biting mom's finger," but mother's intrusive counterreaction perhaps suggests why this is not the case.

With Jane, the depth and richness of some themes were at a fairly superficial level. With the exceptions of building the house and the mildly aggressive interaction with mother, Jane merely described things and materials. During the course of a 50-minute session, one would expect a child of her age and brightness to show a greater capacity for symbolic elaboration and interaction (in contrast to symbolic description). Essentially, she showed that she could describe things in symbolic form by putting words to them, but she did not show, as fully as her potential might indicate, the capacity to elaborate richer fantasies, which one would expect if she were less apprehensive and anxious.

Developmentally, she was focused and engaged, intentional and gesturally interactive, and capable of representational elaboration and differentiation, with, however, significant constrictions.

The sequence of themes was confined to the descriptive level, except for the very interesting sequence where Jane twice used the hand puppets to attack mother and, in the first such attempt, mother quickly took the puppet from her and attacked back. Mother's response was perhaps quite telling; not only was it the only interactive theme, but it was also the only time when both showed some hint of affect over and above the shared apprehensive quality. The constrictions were, therefore, not only in certain affect realms, but in affective, as compared with cognitive, interactions as a whole.

With regard to my subjective reactions, I was impressed with the fact that mother worked so steadily and diligently with Jane and, at the nonaffective level, seemed very responsive to what Jane was doing. She picked up on and reverbalized each of Jane's communications as well as trying to help her construct a "bigger Lego set," build a house, name letters, and so forth. There was a kind of obsessive but very interested and hardworking quality to mother. At the same time, I was as impressed with mother's lack of affect range as I was with Jane's.

Nevertheless, I felt more relaxed and involved, almost like a member of the family, when I sat with them on the floor. It was this feeling that suggested to me that I was probably seeing as much relaxation as this dyad was able to achieve; it also opened a glimpse into the deeper underpinnings of warmth that existed between Jane and her mother, which were perhaps hampered by the chronic apprehension and anxiety they seemed to share. My reaction to mother quickly turning the tables when Jane, in a not terribly belligerent way, attempted to attack her was that mother's quick trigger may be the way she responds to any assertiveness or aggression from Jane.

In sum, Jane was functioning at an age-appropriate level, except in terms of the depth and richness of both her affects and her thematic development. It should be pointed out, however, that both child and mother showed considerable strength in their abilities to focus and concentrate on the task at hand, but would likely have challenges in negotiating assertiveness, anger, and more generally any intense feelings.

CASE 16

Interview

Sam presented as a good-sized, shy 3-year-old who hid behind his mother as he walked somewhat clumsily into the playroom. I suggested they might play together. He was clearly being coy with me, glancing at me occasionally, but then hiding behind his mother.

As soon as he came into the playroom, he tried to get mother to leave with him and pulled at the door. He looked at me. Meanwhile, mother was a little tense and intrusive, putting a puppet in his face and talking quickly; as she made the puppet kiss him, he was trying to push it away. Then he grabbed her leg and held on. As she sat down he clumsily crawled away from her, coming back again and again and hugging and grabbing her. I noticed that he seemed to enjoy crawling over her and hiding behind her to avoid looking at me.

Next, he got up and tried to open a drawer and figure out how it worked. He tried the different things on the drawer and seemed to have an interest in mechanical things. He again looked at me quickly and then looked away.

Mother handed him a ball and he took it. She mentioned that he could throw the ball; he threw it down with a smile. When he threw it a second time, really hard, he had a gleeful look on his face. Mother said, "Oh," and he said "Oh, oh" back. They exchanged "Oh's" as he threw the ball. Next, as he was throwing the ball, she called his name; he ignored her. Sometimes he seemed to "close the circle" and respond to her gestures or vocalizations with gestures or sounds (no words) back, and at other times he didn't respond to her.

Mother tended to intrude and change what he was playing with. If he was throwing a ball, she would try to pick up a doll to get a new activity going, instead of moving in and throwing the ball back. She didn't try to add vocalizations and complexity to the ball throwing. There was always lots of physical contact in her play. She zoomed cars up and down his body to get him to respond. Sam would usually look at her, sometimes seemed to push her away, and at other times began crawling all over her as she moved the cars up and down his body. They exchanged grunts and "Ohs" and high-pitched noises. There was gestural recognition of each other as well as a sense of warmth and connectedness, but they rarely exchanged complex gestures. There were no spontaneous exchanges of words. He persisted in hiding from me, but intermittently looked at me coyly.

When Sam tried to leave the room, he and his mother played with the door. He opened it and she would close it. He would look at her and angrily push it open, and then she would push it closed with a smile. He would then make some sounds and push it open again. This was an organized interaction, but at a simple gestural level. Then, with an abrupt change of pace, mother said, "Let's play ring-around-the-rosie." She grabbed his hand and started dancing with him. She said, "Ring-around-the-rosie," and he, as though they had practiced, would say, "Fall," and they would fall down together. This was their only combined verbal and gestural interaction. He would finish ring-around-the-rosie and make some interactive gestures of a more complex nature as he fell down. At one point, mother tried to help him draw. He fisted the crayon and scribbled chaotically.

As the session evolved, mother got more playful and warm and supportive in her interactions and a little less intrusive and anxious. She indicated to me, as she was playing with him, that at home he sometimes said, "Come now" when he wanted to go somewhere.

I then suggested to mother that she might try to "close as many circles as she could." I explained that opening and closing a circle of communication was when Sam would do A, she would do a B related to his A, and then see if she could encourage him to do a C related to her B. If he could build on her response, he was "closing a circle of communication." They began playing with a toy house with many doors, compartments, and slides. At first mother just sat quietly. She appeared perplexed as to how to join the play. Sam was opening doors and exploring them with good concentration. Then, after he opened the house door, mother handed him a truck. He put the truck in the house and made some sounds and took a truck that had been in the house and gave it to mother. Sam and his mother opened and closed a circle of communication. Mother helped Sam interact while going in the direction he wanted to, rather than distracting, overwhelming, or exciting him. He then continued to examine the house, opening each door. He put dolls in one or the other, understanding clearly how the different slides within the house worked—if he put a doll in one hole, it would come out another hole. As he examined the house, mother and Sam closed some nice gestural circles together; she handed him things that he put in the various compartments, or she caught the dolls as they came out of the compartments and he would hold his hand out for her to return the doll. Their play had a more rhythmic and related quality and they exchanged more sounds together.

Comments

Sam, as suggested by the way he examined the different aspects of the house, could intermittently focus his attention. He was warmly engaged with mother. The quality of warm engagement had a seductive overtone to it on both sides, with lots of physical hugging and handling. When it came to interacting, however, his repertoire was more limited. He was capable of simple gestural interactions, such as taking a toy from mother and putting it into a compartment in the toy house, or indicating and pointing at the office door, and even trying to open it, while making vocal and facial gestures. He did not, however, evidence any complex gestures by stringing together three or four gestures in a row, or doing complex imitations.

The one exception to this was when he played "ring-around-the-rosie, all fall down." He evidenced some minimal use of words, in a gestural sense. His use of a word was not to convey a complex symbolic meaning, but a simple intention.

His mood varied from excited to sober with little joy or happiness. He responded to limits in a variable fashion, but was never out of control. As indicated, there was no evidence of representational (symbolic) play or true representational (verbal) communication.

In terms of developmental patterns, he evidenced scatter in the 12- to 24-month-old range, with most of his gestural and behavioral patterns being suggestive of the 10- to 16-month-old range (the early gestural level). Sam was able to organize himself around simple focused tasks, such as examining the house and its various compartments. He also could organize himself around being shy or being negative. Even at the gestural level, however, he didn't evidence a range of affects or behaviors. There was evidence of curiosity (how the house worked) and assertiveness, explorativeness, and intentionality (e.g., getting mother to hand him the dolls), and gestures were used to convey warmth and closeness with mother. There wasn't happiness, eagerness, or joy. There wasn't the kind of infectious charm that would bring others into his play. Even at the early simple gestural level, he seemed to be constricted, although not severely so. While lacking complex gestural and representational capacities, he showed hints that his level of awareness and his comprehension of his world might be higher than his expressive capacities. This was suggested by the way he took in a new situation, organized his pattern of shyness, and examined how things worked. In his ability to comprehend spatial and mechanical relationships, there were suggestions of circumscribed areas of higher functioning.

In summary, in terms of relating, concentrating, mood, affects, anxiety, and thematic organization, Sam was significantly below age expectations.

CASE 17

Interview

Mother had been thinking of an evaluation for some time for Leah, 25 months of age, because, as mother described immediately upon coming into the office, "She has always been negative and overly sensitive." She explained that it had gotten worse in the last few months after a little brother was born. Also, "She is waking three and four times during the night and isn't happy during the day. She walks around with a solemn, sad look on her face." In addition, "She is always testing and trying to get me to yell at her. I always felt like I was doing something wrong and could never get her to be happy." Mother gave an example in which, at the beach recently, Leah would be happy for 10 minutes, but then be in tears over something—the sand castle wasn't quite right or the food wasn't quite right or mother took too long to get to her, etc. Mother described her as strong willed, wanting it "now" or even "a few minutes before she even asked for it." Father, who also came in, didn't add any comments.

At other times, mother said Leah evidenced gifted intelligence, was verbal, and could sometimes be happy when playing with a little friend. She loved to be read to and could enjoy herself in the sandbox. Occasionally, they could have nice walks together.

After these initial comments, I asked mother and Leah if they would like to play together. I indicated that we could talk more later about Leah's history. Mother was somewhat tense and there was very little sense of emotion coming from her during the play; her gestures and affect expressions seemed empty. She went through the motions, but it gave me the feeling of being in a room where the people had a very mechanical quality to them. Leah looked at me as much as she looked at mother, but with no real joy. Leah was involved in pretend play and was obviously a bright and verbal youngster who could talk in three- or four-word sentences. She was, nonetheless, very solemn looking and marching more to her own drummer than interacting with mother.

At first, she made a little doll go down the slide. Mother, somewhat blandly, asked, "What happens next?" Leah looked back at mother, obviously gesturing her understanding of mother's comment, but then didn't follow up with any verbal comment of her own; she looked back to her doll and the slide and then got hold of a big house and said, "I want to put the people in there."

Leah continued to "tune out" her mother, who would let long periods of silence go by while looking puzzled and somewhat paralyzed with anxiety. Only after a long pause did mother try to comment constructively about what her daughter wanted to do with the people in the house. By that time, Leah was already beginning to look around the room for additional toys to bring into her emerging drama. Leah continued her methodical, vaguely organized play, occasionally using elaborate descriptions, such as, "Now I am going to have the dolls try to find a horsey for them to ride." Mother looked on passively in silence, neither jumping to help her find a horsey or showing interest in what the dolls were going to do on the horsey. After a pregnant pause of about 10 seconds, she tried to follow Leah's lead by saying, "Gee, do they want other animals, too?" Leah ignored mother, looking at her as though to say with a solemn, angry look, "Too little, too late."

Father, who had been very quiet, then got down on the floor and started playing with Leah. Father, in contrast to mother, was intrusive, rather than avoidant or laid-back. As father started manipulating Leah's dolls and the horses and other animals (she had gathered them together for the dolls to ride), he said, "Oh, I think they are going to go here and I think they are going to go there." He had an enthusiastic and aggressive look. His play had a somewhat anxious, clumsy, intrusive quality. Leah then said adamantly, with clear annoyance in her voice, "They are my toys!" and pulled his fingers off the toys. Father then jumped back in. The next 10 minutes were characterized by Leah turning her back to him and trying to push him away, and father trying to push himself into her play. They actually had quite a few interactions around the theme of him intruding and her pushing him away. As father got discouraged, he became more active and then tried to engage in some "horsing around," where he tried to pick her up and throw her up in the air and have her jump on his tummy. She squirmed away from him and somewhat angrily screeched and got back to her toys. He was not able to get into a comfortable rhythm with her and vacillated between attempting physical play, being overintrusive, and occasionally having a few minutes when he just observed and seemed to regroup.

Next, I got down on the floor and played with Leah. I noted that she was quite capable of engaging in contingent and reciprocal interactions. I joined her theme of trying to get the different dolls on the horses. She seemed to take charge of the drama, but accepted my assistance. As I handed her dolls, she looked at me, and occasionally nodded her head. When I asked, "What next?" she would explain that the horses were going to go over here, or that this doll was going to go on the horse next, or this doll was going on the horse after that. Her verbal, elaborative productions were responsive to my simple comments or questions; her gestures were elaborating on mine and the interactions were clearly related to one another. She was able to operate on a simple "pretend" level. There were no "buts" or "becauses" or elaborate themes. The themes stayed pretty much around getting the dolls on the horses and seeing where the horses would go. During the representational interactions there was a sense of relatedness. She could limit impulses. Even when she got frustrated with the doll not being able to do what she wanted it to, she didn't bang or throw the horse, but simply tried again. Her mood was even during these efforts.

She was easily able to organize a number of units of representation into a reasonably long sequence—the theme of the dolls and horses. At the same time, however, her emotional range was quite limited; she looked serious and sad. She occasionally showed some annoyance when the horse or the doll wouldn't do what she wanted it to do. There were no signs of pleasure or joy, or of her broadening her themes. No themes of warmth and closeness emerged other than her general sense of relatedness.

Comments

Leah was an organized, intentional child capable of complex intentional behavior and gestures. She could use short intentional sentences. She was engaged with me and her parents, and capable of beginning representational play and interactions. At the same time, she was serious and sad, lacking pleasure, joy, and spontaneity.

Leah's parents had difficulty engaging her in a broad range of representational or prerepresentational interactions. The most striking aspects of mother's involvement were mother's emptiness, her lack of joyful affect, and her tendency toward long pauses. In contrast, the interactions with father were characterized by his intrusive style; Leah was constantly fending him off. Both parents could be logical and organized. One parent seemed to be leaving Leah empty while the other seemed to be trying to control and overload her.

She could focus, relate, interact intentionally, and use representational modes for organizing experience. But her mood was sober and her affect range was limited (little joy or spontaneity). Her thematic overtures were around issues of controlling the action, making sure the dolls and people were doing things her way.

CASE 18

Interview

Mother, a 39-year-old attorney, came alone to the first session to talk about Elizabeth, who was 3½ months old. She quickly told me, "I have a feeling that my baby doesn't like me. She doesn't look at me. I feel incompetent and helpless. After my baby was born, I felt that others could do it better, almost like I felt when I was trying my first case—others could do it better than me." Mother added, "I look at her and I feel sad when she isn't looking back at me."

Mother was 39 years old when she had her baby; "Life was fleeting by," she said. "Now I can look at her sometimes and feel how cute she is and it gives my life meaning. But I also worry that she's not looking at me." She described Elizabeth as a "sweet and

placid baby," while reiterating that she had a baby nurse for the first
2 months. "I was an only child," she explained. "I needed to plunge
in, to learn how to be a mommy, but didn't do it. Now I feel awkward
and uncomfortable." Mother reported that she hired a nanny, a woman
in her late 40s, who she hoped would help her feel more confident.
Elizabeth's father was a stockbroker who worked hard and didn't get
home until 7:30 or 8:00 P.M. Mother hoped to get back to working
hard again soon as well.

As mother talked, with tight control of her face and vocal
tone, she seemed passive and cautious, often feeling helpless and
empty. There was a sense that she needed to be filled up and was
finding it hard to fill anyone else up. This quality was conveyed even
in the way she reached out with her words. Her affect was constricted.
Her thinking was organized but somewhat concrete; she would not
elaborate on the few details she mentioned. At the same time, she
seemed to have a desire to be reflective and to figure things out.

She went on to reveal that she had always been scared of
taking care of other people, even as a babysitter. As early as fourth
grade, "I was always afraid of death and dying and that bad things
would happen if I took care of people."

At the second meeting, mother brought Elizabeth in with her.
Elizabeth was a small 3½-month-old baby who didn't look at either
her mother or me, except for a fleeting second here and there. If
mother persisted in talking to her, she did respond with an occasional
fleeting look toward mother's voice, but there were no robust smiles.
Mother was very tentative in the way she interacted with Elizabeth,
whispering in a kind of monotone, rather than varying her pitch and
pulling Elizabeth in. She held her stiffly and anxiously at a distance.
I also noticed that as mother interacted with Elizabeth, she got discouraged easily. She would pause for a few seconds longer than one
would expect, flattening her rhythm so that even if she had Elizabeth's
attention for a second, she couldn't vary her pitch to hold it. Mother
would often go silent for 5 or 6 seconds and then start up again in a
tense whisper. She hardly varied her facial expression or the way she
held Elizabeth—about 8 inches from her and with stiff, rigid hands
around her abdomen and back, as if this was how she had seen it
done in a textbook. The atmosphere between the two of them was
one of an eerie kind of tension. It lacked warmth and feeling. Elizabeth
either stared off at the wall or looked fleetingly past her mother.

When I tried to interact with Elizabeth, she came comfortably
into my lap, without any fuss or change in her facial expression. She
had good motor tone, perhaps a bit higher than expected. At one
point as I was talking to her, she got a little fussy, but calmed easily
when I put her on my shoulder and applied gentle pressure to her

back. As I played with her and stroked her arms and legs gently, I didn't notice any smiles, nor were there any aversive signs—no head-turning away or look of discomfort—both with light touch to arms, legs, abdomen, and back and with firm pressure in those areas. I worked with her, making interesting facial expressions and moving my head back and forth, and noticed that she responded a little better, in terms of following my face, when I was very animated. I also noted that she liked to look at one toy in particular. When I spoke to her, I noticed that she focused a little less well on my voice. If I was very persistent and varied my pitch only slightly from one second to the next, giving her a slowly changing pattern, she could begin to focus more, going from perhaps from 1 second to 2½ seconds. When I made sounds with her fingers she blinked, grimaced, or tensed up for a second. She therefore had a rather fleeting pattern of joint attention with me. She would focus from 1 to 2½ seconds and then tune out and look at a lamp or something else around the room. Occasionally she had a faint, beginning grin on her face, but no broad, robust smiles.

Elizabeth was patient with me during the 15 minutes or so I worked with her. She didn't get upset or fussy as I tried laying her on her back on my lap, had her do sit-ups with me holding her hands, and held her in front of me; her fleeting attention was consistent in all positions. She would do best when I combined very animated facial expressions with a very slowly changing vocal rhythm. If the vocal rhythm became too fast or monotonous like mother's, I could only hold her attention for about a second. She did not enjoy brisk movement in space, but preferred very slow rhythmic movements, both horizontally and vertically. She also seemed to enjoy slow, rhythmic rocking rather than very rapid movements, which tended to startle her.

Comments

It appeared from this first session with Elizabeth that she was having difficulty reaching the first milestone of shared attention and forming a relationship (engagement). She was finding it hard to tune into vocalizations, doing slightly better with visual experiences. She appeared to be a little hyporeactive in the area of processing vocal experience. She was also mildly sensitive to brisk movement in space. Her response to touch and her motor tone, though, seemed appropriate. Therefore, she seemed to be a laid-back type of baby who was a little hyporeactive, requiring lots of wooing and work. Yet, she was also sensitive to loud noises and movement in space. Coupled with these individual differences, Elizabeth's mother was a very tense, anxious person who could provide little visual or vocal/verbal experimentation to find the right rhythms to engage Elizabeth. Mother also felt easily rejected and empty, almost requiring, as she put it, "a baby who could fill me up." Mother was also worried that she was somehow "bad." In some respects, Elizabeth fitted the description mother had given of herself as a child—someone who was waiting for the other person to woo her. We therefore had a situation where Elizabeth's individual differences and mother's individual differences were making the early phase of shared attention and engagement hard to negotiate.

Elizabeth required certain types of experience geared to her individual differences, and mother would need some help to learn how to interact with Elizabeth in the narrow "pathway" that Elizabeth found comfortable.

5

Conducting the Interview

THE PURPOSE OF the diagnostic interview can be stated simply—to learn as much as possible about the child. The interviewer's basic task, therefore, is to create a setting that maximizes the amount of information that can be observed. As you conduct the interview, ask yourself what you can do to create a richer learning experience, in particular, what would evoke more data relevant to the categories that we have been discussing or to other categories that you may have constructed. A subsidiary goal is to establish rapport with the child so he or she will not feel frightened about returning for future visits if treatment or further diagnostic sessions are indicated. Let us begin with some general perspectives and principles and then talk about the opening phase, the middle phase, and the ending phase of the interview.

Training yourself to be a skillful observer is essential to the conduct of a successful interview. Related to this is evolving a personally comfortable style. There are two basic approaches—the structured and the unstructured interview. Briefly, the structured interview consists of using techniques that direct the child toward certain play materials and then asking certain questions. An older child may be asked about his or her family, while a younger child may be asked to fill in the endings of certain stories.

Many of you are familiar with the "baby bird" story: the interviewer starts it by saying that a baby bird falls out of the nest, and the child is asked to finish the story. Another well-known example begins with the question, If you had three wishes, what would they be? In other words, as in sentence-completion tests, you start the child off with certain ambiguous or semidirected stimuli and the child is asked to complete them.

You may also structure the interview with devices of your own, for example, greeting the child in a certain way or posing a question about dreams. Whatever structure you employ, however, it is important to bear in mind that the child is responding to what you are doing, and you must observe and understand his or her reaction in this context. As you gain experience with many children, you will get a sense of the average range of expectable responses to the structured elements you employ. You will also learn to understand individual differences in response to the kinds of issues that you may raise.

The unstructured interview, in contrast to the above approach, follows the basic concept that the less you intrude, the more the child will tell you. I favor the unstructured approach because I think it creates more of a learning opportunity. Structure tends to contaminate your observations and makes it hard to know how much of what is going on is a product of what you are doing and how much is what the child is bringing to the situation. For a variety of reasons that are not altogether clear, most children will , if given the chance, let you know what is going on in their personality—both structurally, in terms of how well they can handle reality testing, impulse control, and the like, and experientially, in terms of thoughts, fantasies, and feelings.

Your primary interest, I need hardly add, lies in observing whatever material the child is willing to share with you. The advantage of the unstructured interview is that it allows children to tell their stories in their own way, which is equivalent to saying that it allows children to put their own structure on the situation. There will be ample opportunity to get responses to structured stimuli via psychological testing and discussions with parents and teachers.

An unstructured interview may seem to have more potential for what you may consider mistakes. Remember, the interview is an interactive process, not a series of isolated comments. Your thoughtful comments or gestures, even ones that, in retrospect, you may feel were not quite perfectly timed or optimally empathetic, lead to a reaction on the part of the child. If you observe the nature of that reaction, you can then use it constructively in that child's interest. In the remainder of this chapter I will explain how to conduct an unstructured interview.

Two general principles for the clinician's conduct during the interview will be suggested: 1) the clinician must tolerate his or her own discomfort as well as that of the patient to permit the full extent of the psychopathology to emerge, and 2) the clinician should observe continually in all the categories describes in Chapter 2.

The specific principles for the beginning, middle, and end of the interview will also be suggested: 1) During the initial phase, be warm and accepting, but not too seductive or charming in order to permit patients to show you (with minimal interference from you) how they begin a new relationship and what their own perceptions or anticipations are for this new experience (e.g., expecting to be exploited and humiliated, stuck with needles, filled up with good candy and cake, sexually seduced, competed with). 2) During the middle phase of the interview, facilitate patients' associative trends and observe the organization, depth, richness, and sequence of affects, themes, sense of relatedness, mood, etc. Comments from the perspective of the patient's ego and sense of mastery may be useful with regard to his or her initial perception of the meaning of the interview (especially if it is fearful) as well as in dealing with conflicts and/or themes or affects that may emerge during the middle phase of the interview. In essence, the goal of the middle phase is to help patients permit you "to get to know them," and to observe this process carefully, noting how much patients facilitate the goal on their own and how they use your help (e.g., ignore your comments, get disorganized, or use your comments to enrich their associative trends both affectively and thematically). 3) During the last phase of the interview, observe how patients prepare for and deal with separation from you and with your comments on relevant themes, and—most important—how they deal with highly stressful, potentially frightening affects that might undermine future diagnostic or therapeutic work. The goal here is to help patients consolidate, from the perspective of their ego or mastery, a sense of a unique and useful experience.

Before elaborating the basic principles, I want to make a suggestion: use notepaper with columns drawn for each category to facilitate your task of maximum observation; you can then enter your observations in the appropriate columns as the interview progresses. Another method is to make notes that give a running description of the interview, keeping the categories in the back of your mind. After several interviews, observing in all the categories becomes almost automatic. With practice it becomes easy to reconstruct the interview afterward.

Now to the basic principles. To become a good, noninterfering observer, you must follow the principle of tolerating discomfort in the child as well as in yourself. You are not going to be able to diagnose psychopathology unless you permit the child to show it to you. If a child shows anxiety (e.g., by disrupting play or crying) and you move in too quickly to support him rather than letting him play it out for you, you will not observe how well he can handle it on his own. Of course, you always have to make a clinical judgment in these areas. If a child becomes very disorganized and frightened, you may have to move in and help him restructure his world. Symbolically speaking, you do not want the child to hurt once you have observed the nature of the psychopathology. However, you do want to observe fully just how deep and intense that psychopathology is, and this you cannot do if you close off the behavior prematurely.

When the time has come to be supportive, it is best to comment on the behavior rather than gloss over the child's difficulty and shift attention away from it. For example, it is important for 4- and 5-year-olds to feel that you are not only interested in what they tell you but also that you are not frightened by it. When you make a statement in an area of difficulty, children are often greatly relieved to know that finally they have met someone who is not frightened by what frightens them. Although a child may be too afraid to talk about a problem directly in the first interview, he or she will at least know that you are ready to listen.

As for our own discomfort, there are certain kinds of behavior that cause anxiety in most of us, no matter how experienced we are—for example, primitive disorganized behavior. We like nice garden-variety neurotic conflicts that may be similar to our own and therefore easy to understand. But we dislike and will tend to cut off primitive behavior, particularly if it touches on something in our own unconscious. Often we do not recognize our own anxiety as such. Instead, we may experience a first-level defense against it, which might very well be the thought, "This child is getting too disorganized. I'd better structure the interview for her." What one really may be thinking is, "Her behavior or feelings make me too disorganized. I had better structure the interview for myself." If, in the first diagnostic interview, you feel the need to move in very quickly, your first thought should be, am I taking care of myself or am I taking care of this child? Far more than adults, children possess a marvelous talent for touching on our own sensitive areas, probably because they wear their conflicts much more on their sleeves, so to speak. With children, our own countertransference or reaction tendencies will be much more easily elicited. If you find yourself becoming uncomfortable, it is best to say nothing, observe what happens for at least a few minutes, and note any fantasies of your own that come to mind.

The next principle is the one I have been elaborating all along, that is, follow the communications of the child—not only the content of the themes, but also the associative trends from the viewpoint of the child's relatedness, emotional tone, and affects over time. Also follow the child in terms of developmental levels. Is she engaged and focused, using gestures to communicate intentionally and to negotiate basic issues in the relationship? Is she able to elaborate affects and emotional themes in a representational form using either words or pretend play? Or is motor discharge and only descriptive use of language her way of relating? Is she able to differentiate her representations with categories and build bridges between them? Or is she fragmented or shallow? For which emotional themes is she capable of more or less advanced levels of organizing experience? Describe, for example, disengagement around anger. This principle will be further exemplified as the different phases of the interview are discussed below.

The first phase of the interview begins in the waiting room. Your first observations are of the child with his or her parents; notice their spatial relationship and interactions. Then, as discussed in Chapter 2, before approaching the parents or child, pause for a moment and get your first impressions of the child, noticing such things as physical makeup, coordination, gross and fine motor activity, and sensory motor functioning. Observe how the child responds to mother and other family members, as well as to other people in the room. You may even have an opportunity to see gestures, affects, and activities that give you information for some of the other categories.

For example, you may begin to see a range of emotion as the child navigates the room. You may observe a moment of stress between the child and mother if the child is disobedient. This interaction will allow you to observe how the child handles anxiety. If the child is playing alone or with another person you can even see something of his or her thematic organization and range. Clearly, the observations in those first few minutes in the waiting room need to be supplemented with additional material from the interview, but they can provide you with an initial impression of the child's status in many of the developmental categories and with a preliminary intuitive feeling for the child.

As for beginning your interaction, it is preferable to make contact with the child before doing so with the parents if the child seems available to you. In this way, the child begins to understand that you are mainly interested in getting to know him or her. After your greeting, simply ask the child to come with you to the playroom. Here again, there will be some interesting behavior to observe as the child begins relating to you as a new person. If you just offer them your person without any seductive, sugar-coated trimmings, most healthy children will show some trepidation, some mild apprehension, some mild caution, yet a trusting-enough attitude to come along with you because they usually have some sense about why they are there. If, on the other hand, you approach the child with cookies or candies, you will not get a picture of the ordinary way this particular child responds to a new person.

Some children may run ahead of you when you point to the room. Others will lag a few feet behind you. If the child is very young, you may offer your hand. You will get an intuitive sense of when to do that. Other children may refuse to leave mother, and your first diagnostic task may be how to deal with the child who is holding on to mother and refusing to separate. In some such cases you may want to take a step back and see what mother or father does. Some parental figures will grab little Sally, saying, "You've got to go into the room, you are embarrassing me," and then take the child by the arm and drag her into the room. Although you feel motivated to interfere because you think the parents are being brutal to the child, I think you are wiser to wait and see how the parent deals with the child and how the child deals with the parent: does the child provoke the mother, for instance, or is it the other way around? In any case, you can assume that if the parent behaves that way here, he or she does so everywhere. At a certain point you may want to do something to ease the situation, but it is useful to get the natural picture first. Do not let your own anxiety interfere with your observing the situation for a short time.

I usually have the playroom set up with toys or games appropriate to the child's age so that the room is somewhat organized when the youngster enters. I welcome children with a warm hello and a smile and then let them make the first move. Some people believe in giving candy to establish a bond between the therapist and child; however, I regard this as a spurious gift because the therapist has something much better—professional skill—to offer. Once the child senses this, he or she will relate to the therapist in a far more profound way than through a gift of candy. I do not ask, "Do you know why you are here?" because it limits the potential range of responses the child may show. For instance, in response to this direct question the following dialogue may ensue.

C: Because my mother said I should come.
T: Why did your mother say you should come?
C: I don't know.
T: Oh, come on, you know.
C: No, I don't know.
T: Oh, come on, your mother must have told you something.
C: Well, it has something to do with school. I don't do well in school.
T: Why don't you do well in school?
C: Well, I don't know and I am not going to tell you!

This is not an uncharacteristic interview with a child. Although there is nothing wrong with having such an exchange, you do not learn as much as you would if you allowed the child to tell you in his own way (and he will) why he thinks he is there.

With reference to the situation you and the child are about to share, you can be sure that he has a preconceived notion of why he is there and how he is going to handle it. If you explain too quickly who you are, how long you are going to be together, etc., you will not learn what the child's ideas are. Similarly, although you may have the benefit of the child's history from the parents, you should not confront the child with this material, for it may elicit the response, "If that is what they told you, why don't you talk to them about it." However, you certainly should use the information (symptoms) related by the parents as one perspective from which to observe the child. For example, if the parents have told you that the child is stealing, you might watch for signs of emotional hunger—that is, does the child steal in order to "fill himself up," or for signs of anger— does the child steal in retaliation? You might also be alert to sneaky or tricky maneuvers, a derivation of stealing.

Once the child has shared with you as many of his perceptions as he is able to, you should give him some feedback on what he has told you to show that you understand. You can also correct any distortions by offering your understanding of his concerns, and you can set out certain terms of your relationship, such as how long you will be together on this occasion and whether you will be seeing him again. Depending on the child's age, you may want to describe how you see the goals of your time together. Once again, you will do well to wait until you have heard the child express his or her goals before stating your own (which should be explained in a context the child will understand). For instance, if a child says that she expects something special, you can explain, "Although I know you want some cake and candy from me, I'm going to try and help you in a different way." That way the child will know that she has been heard and understood.

At this point you may also want to tell the child the rules of the playroom—typically, that he is free to play, and say and do anything he wants, but he cannot break anything or hurt either you or himself. Laying down the rules of the playroom often gives the youngster a sense of freedom. Some children do not appear to need this explanation, as if they intuitively know the rules. Others appear to be frozen until you give them permission to explore, and still others immediately act aggressively. Again, do not explain the rules until you have seen how the child reacts to the room, otherwise you will miss an important piece of information about the child's personality.

The ambiguity present in the first few minutes is almost always an occasion of learning. For instance, one child in that first moment of anxiety looked around the room and asked if there was a tape recorder, a specific concern I might not have heard if I had intruded too quickly.

Another child came in and lay face down on the couch. Waiting to see what he would do, I felt that he was telling me something. Did he want to be in analysis (maybe he has a parent in analysis), was it a sign of dependency, was he terribly tired, or was fear causing him to bury his head like an ostrich? After some moments I described to him what he was doing and wondered if he could tell me what he was feeling about it. It evolved later in the interview that something frightening had happened to him just before the interview. From his behavior, I saw one of the ways he deals with frightening experiences.

Another child, a 9-year-old, began by sitting down in a mature way and telling me that his mother had brought him because he was fighting with his little sister. I got the feeling from his demeanor that he was waiting for something. I commented on this and he said, "Yes, I'm waiting for my shot. When you go to doctors, you get shots." He described this huge needle that I was going to use and went on to say that although his mother said I was a different kind of doctor, not the kind that gave injections, he did not believe her. He still expected a huge shot and he expressed this with an air of excitement. Later on I commented that he had not seemed frightened by the idea of the needle, and this set him off into other areas of expectations that led to a picture of some of his conflicts.

With regard to children who are initially rigid and silent, suppressing your immediate urge to structure their activities will allow you to discover whether such children can begin something on their own. The following examples illustrate this.

A bright 7-year-old came in, sat down on my couch, and looked at me. I looked at him. I let that go on for maybe 30 seconds, which is very long in that situation. Most people would tolerate no more than 5 or 10 seconds before moving in to structure the situation and make it more comfortable. This particular child seemed to become more frozen with anxiety as time went on. When I saw his discomfort growing and realized that he was only going to get more rigid, I ended the silence. I had observed what I wanted to know; that is, I learned that he could not overcome his anxiety, and thus began structuring the situation. By tolerating his discomfort and my own, I learned that he could not take charge, so to speak.

Another child started out exactly the same way, seemingly frozen, but after about 20 seconds she made a comment about the room, relating it to her own house. She continued to make herself comfortable by associating back and forth, essentially saying that being there with me was not all that unfamiliar and frightening to her. Obviously it *is* a new and frightening situation, and this child was demonstrating a tremendous coping capacity that spoke volumes to me about how she deals with a stressful situation.

With children like the one in the first example, I try to say something that picks up on what I think the child is feeling; or if I want to be more impersonal about it, I will say that people sometimes come here (to the interview room) and don't know what to make of the situation. To the silent boy, I said, "You're not sure what to think or say." He then made a few comments about the house we were in that made him feel a little more relaxed. That got him grounded and he said, "I don't know why I'm here or what I'm supposed to do." He wanted me to give him direction.

At that point most 7-year-olds would be opening up the toy closet, looking around the room, exploring the range of options available to them. Therefore, with this particular child I did not immediately accept that he did not know what to do. I said, "You have no idea at all?" and continued with comments about how it feels to be in a strange place with no idea why you are there and what his parents may have told him. Once I broached the latter issue with him, he somewhat reluctantly said, "Well, you're a doctor who talks about feelings." Then he slowly revealed to me that his parents had told him that he was coming to talk about feelings and that they had already talked to me; he added that he felt "strange" about his own feelings. Then we were off and running, but it had taken a good 10 minutes of exploration before he was willing to tell me that he had some understanding—which was fairly profound—of why he was there.

His initial feeling of strangeness, communicated through silence, was indeed where *he* wanted to begin. In the end, I did not have to tell him much of anything. All I had to do was confirm his understanding of the situation. He showed me he was a boy who holds back, who uses a passive stance to life as a way of dealing with a whole variety of issues. (In fact, this was one of the problems his parents were concerned about, that their bright child was not doing well in school and had trouble asserting himself.) I was able to see that behind the passive stance there was a considerable reservoir. Once he got started, he was able to develop well-organized themes and a sense of relatedness to me. He showed me that his passive stance was not a rigid defense covering up some major defects in core personality functioning, for example. I saw that this was a child with many assets who was troubled by "strange feelings."

With respect to making comments, warm affect is important:

what you say is not as crucial as *how* you say it. Above all, in the first few minutes do not begin steering the child in a particular direction. Leave him free to choose an initial theme. You do want to indicate your understanding of his feeling, to give him some feedback on what he has told you, but you do not want to lead him with your comment. By making a supportive comment you are not only telling the child what he is doing, you are showing him what you have to offer. With a challenging child, such as one who is rigid, it is important not to be too easy on him, or you will not learn the answer to some of the difficult differential diagnostic questions.

For example, if you are seductive and appealing, even a seriously depressed child will respond by giving you all sorts of interesting dynamic material. This may help you understand her conflicts but, in so behaving, you may miss the fact that she is depressed or basically negativistic. You may indeed want to use charm at some point in the treatment relationship where it may have particular value in helping the child understand something or helping her ally with you in the observing function. Until such time, however, your comments should be warmly empathic, but not too much so, and never cold or remote, for either extreme will contaminate the child's reaction.

The extreme opposite to the rigid child is the child who is uncontrollable. Here you have to decide when to step in. Let us say you are 5 minutes into the interview and the child is smashing things and beginning to kick you. What you do partly depends on what you are willing to tolerate. Some therapists will tolerate some breakage but will physically try to control the child if they are hit. Others will let the child continue through the whole session in order to see at what point the child will finally feel enough involvement to be able to control himself.

If you feel physical restraint is required, you can try with your gestures to show the seriousness of your limits as you make comments in an effort to calm the child. Bringing in the parents may help the child organize himself. You need to decide, sometimes, if you or the parents should assist the child by holding him if his behavior demands it. I would use the situation to learn about the child and not assume after two or three outbursts that some sort of restraint is necessary. Such a decision is a matter of personal style. Some clinicians are willing to risk more exhaustion than others.

Some of you may find that your own personality is such that difficult children, particularly aggressive ones, tend to get organized in your presence and will not challenge your authority. Others may find that, on the contrary, such children challenge you repeatedly. Some of you may be better with passive children. A frightened and passive child, seeing a person who conveys an image of authority, may withdraw for most of the session. With a less imposing figure, a gentler or more soft-spoken person, that same child may be willing to engage in a dialogue. It is important to know your own baseline and the kinds of reactions that you tend to induce.

You also should know yourself well enough to know the responses certain kinds of children evoke in you. All of us will have different reactions to the same child, and it is important to learn what yours are likely to be. If you are uncomfortable with aggression, you may react paradoxically with sympathy and pity toward aggressive children. Although you may work well therapeutically with them, it is important to know that your idiosyncratic reaction to these aggressive children is to feel extraordinarily "maternal." You want to make them "nice" children, to overlook or excuse their aggressiveness. You see only the needy and deprived side rather than seeing this together with the aggressive side. The point is not that you should change your reaction but rather that you should learn how to use it. Then it becomes another instrument, another source of information for you.

Some children will not be verbal or even use pretend play. You should have no difficulty in being available for presymbolic communication. The child still has a lot to tell you. He focuses and engages or he is aloof and removed. His gestures are random and aimless or he is quite intentional and organized in the way he smiles, vocalizes, points, stands or sits, looks, grimaces, etc. Does he use gestures to negotiate certain emotional themes and become more aimless and disengaged with others (e.g., aimless around dependency and organized around anger)? The child who, because of a language or cognitive delay or for emotional reasons, operates in a presymbolic mode may reveal more to you in a direct fashion that will help you figure out his patterns than his symbolic counterpart. Remember, always try to engage and communicate with the child at his level, even while you may be trying to encourage higher levels of communication. For example, with the gesturing child, use animated gestures together with your words.

In summary, during the first phase of the interview you should be concerned with the child communicating why he is there, how he views you, and how he understands the situation. While this part of the child's story is unfolding, it is important not to direct his thoughts or activities. The comments you make during the first phase of the interview should show your supportive understanding of the child's concerns. Your comments should clarify the goals of the session once the child has shared his notions of why he is seeing you, and they should serve to establish a working relationship between you and the child, that is, show the child that you can understand and help him.

The middle phase of the interview offers excellent opportunities to observe in all the categories discussed in Chapter 2. By this time the child will have evinced some predominant affects, begun to form some kind of relationship with you, shown you an overall emotional tone, and developed a theme that probably had some disruptions in it, allowing you the opportunity to see the child handle anxiety. You will be noting the thematic sequences, which help to create linkages, as well as the richness, depth, and age-appropriateness of the themes, which tell you something about the structural capacities of the child's personality. During this time, it is also important to note your own subjective reactions and fantasies.

The major goal of the middle phase of the interview is to facilitate the unfolding of the child's story. You want to follow his leads and help him make associative links when his own defenses create a block. The preconscious and unconscious elements of the story will emerge in terms of the sequence as the child moves from theme to theme. The job of the diagnostician is to make sense of what may seem like a series of disjointed themes. By listening with a sensitive ear, one can follow the trend of associations. With an adult this is done through understanding a series of statements; with a child it is achieved by observing the evolution of play, words, affect, gestures, and relatedness to you throughout the interview.

After you get a picture of how well the child can organize themes, you can make comments that help the child find transition points or linkages. Basically, your comments should try to play back the theme that the child has presented. It may be quite difficult at times to pinpoint the theme because of the complex ways in which children communicate: the meanings conveyed through play, body posture, and style of relating can be exceedingly subtle. Your comments should also focus on whatever category seems most immediate or relevant to a particular child. With some children you may want to comment on the affect—for example, "It seems like people feel angry a lot." Or you may want to comment on the story line—for example, "It seems like every time people get close, they lose the people that they care for." Let us say the child is dealing with jealousy and is markedly anxious and tense. A helpful comment might be: "You know, when people want a lot and there is only a little bit, sometimes people get very nervous and tense." In this case your comment focused on the content and affect.

Because our categories of observation are all integral parts of a child's internal economy—all parts of the way she experiences her world—you cannot go too far off the mark no matter which category you choose to emphasize. Still, if you are able to comment on the area of most intense involvement, the child will probably respond better and develop her communications more fully and richly. Make your comments curious rather than provocative. Even a "Tell me more about that" will help. In general, if a child is stuck (i.e, repetitive) at the level of content, you may want to highlight the affect, and vice versa.

When making comments, it is especially important to be aware of another general principle, that is, try not to ask questions. Put whatever you need to say in the form of a declarative statement. If a child is behaving aggressively toward you, instead of asking, "Are you angry with me?" or "Do you tend to get angry?" say to him or her, "It seems that you are angry," "You are trying to hurt me," and so on. Making such statements also suggests to the child that putting things into words is another way of expressing thoughts and feelings. This gives the child another option, one with more flexibility than wordless action or internal fantasy.

It is important to stay away from comments directly oriented toward increasing any fearful, instinctually laden impulses you may observe. Although you should recognize the child's frightening thoughts and feelings, stay on the side of the child that is trying to master her fears. Let us say a child is nearly overwhelmed with all kinds of instinctually laden wishes and fears of what might happen, but consciously feels panicked and confused. To say, "This must be a confusing situation," is to address the conscious part of her ego, the side of her personality that actively processes experience. Even this comment may be threatening, however. The child may be one who is easily humiliated; she may respond by showing you how strong she is, saying, "No, I never get confused about anything." Then you will recover quickly by saying, "It seems as though it's best to be in control of things. You like to be on top of things." Here, instead of using charged phrases such as, "You don't like to be helpless . . . passive . . . humiliated," you say, "You like to be in charge of things . . . in control." Usually the child will agree with you. At first you will not know which are the charged words, but after you make some initial comments, you will begin to sense which words to stay away from, and will be better equipped to phrase supportive comments.

For example, suppose a child tells you about other children on the block who like to beat up people, then suddenly goes silent and starts spinning around and moving rhythmically. You see the child's anxiety has gotten high, causing her to regress to rhythmical body movements. At that point you might say, "Gee, talking about people beating up other people is a scary kind of thing." Now that may either help the child to go on or she may choose not to tell you anything else about beating up people. She may switch to drawing or something else less affectively laden, and then come back to the theme of aggression later on. By pointing out to her that it is frightening to talk about angry feelings (she showed you how frightening she found it by switching to a rhythmic type of behavior pattern right after mentioning it), you are showing the child that you can understand and accept her concerns and that you know they are frightening; thus you are not siding solely with the drive component of her revelation. One does not say, "Tell me more about aggression," but instead sides in a balanced way with both the coping capacity and the affects and drives that cause anxiety.

Another example is provided by the child who gets caught up in repeatedly punching the Bobo doll and the beanbag after taking off the doll's clothing. After you have observed how he integrates the theme of punching and anger with other aspects of the playroom, as well as how he relates to you and what kind of affects are generated, you might move in and say something quite simple, e.g., "You know, punching and taking off clothes both seem to be very important to you." With this comment you may help the child extend his associations, thereby getting a picture of his willingness to deepen and enrich his themes.

At some point around the middle of the interview, if you feel you have a sense of what the child is communicating, it is sometimes helpful to pull together a number of elements into what might be called an "ego-related clarification" (not synonymous with an interpretation). Such a clarifying statement would include the affects that are manifested, the key thematic material accompanying these affects, and the way the child is dealing with these elements. The child's reaction to the clarification can teach you a good deal about how he organizes his thinking and deals with conflict-ridden material.

As with simpler comments, the manner in which the clarification is offered is important to its success. The clarification should side with the child's ego rather than trying to interpret deep unconscious longings, hungers, or aggressive feelings. You should always maintain a balance, seeing the coping capacity as well as the underlying wishes and fears, but have that balance lean toward the child's strengths.

For example, suppose that during the first half of the interview the child has demonstrated anger, jealousy, and rage and shown little of the compassionate and empathic affects. Using dolls, he has been unfolding a story in which his schoolmates mistreat him and think they are better than he is. Later he plays out the same story with the toy animals and has a policeman step in to stop their fighting. He continues to repeat this theme in a controlled way without developing it further. You ask him to tell you more about the fighting, hoping that he will make the theme deeper and richer. Instead he replays it in a more obsessive way, showing you the issue of control.

You decide to make a clarification based on the affect and the story line. You say how important it is to be in control of things when people feel angry, hoping that the child will use the clarification to reach a deeper level of association. He becomes provocative and counterphobic, taking a gun and shooting darts at you. You make another clarification, again reflecting on his wishes, themes, and styles of coping: "Yes, sometimes when people feel unsure of being able to control their feelings, one way to deal with it is to attack." Reassured because he sees that you have understood him, the child now begins further exploration of the underlying issues, which I regard as a good prognostic sign for the child in treatment.

In all cases, you want to watch closely how a child responds to your clarifications. The behavior may be indirect; the child may move to another part of the room and start a new activity such as drawing. But while the child is drawing, you may suddenly realize that through this activity he or she is indeed telling you more about aggressive feelings or fears of separation. You see that the child has essentially taken in and integrated your comments and moved onto another plane, thus offering you a greater understanding of what is going on. The clarification has given the child a beginning sense of what therapy can be, a sense that a trained person can help the child organize things in a way that he or she could not do alone.

At the midway point of the interview you will have done much of the important work: observed how the child develops themes and relates to you, noted where different affects are demonstrated, and so on. You have given the child the opportunity to tell you what is on his mind and how he is feeling about life in general, and you have made clarifications and watched his reactions to them. While offering helpful comments as needed, continue to observe how the child develops his story, all the while watching for increasing depth and range in the seven categories.

As the end of the session nears, begin to summarize the important issues the child has been communicating to you. Such comments, which convey to the child the fact that your meeting will soon end, will allow you to see how he or she deals with separation. Keep in mind that any shifts in behavior may be related to the expected separation. Thus, a well-modulated child may suddenly start being aggressive, and a somewhat withdrawn child may start coming closer, even clinging to you. A child who has been quiet during most of the interview may finally show a willingness to talk about feelings, perhaps rousing your anxiety because you feel must extend the interview time. However, you must realize that the child's very motive in opening up may be to keep you involved so that he or she does not have to leave. In such a situation you might say, "Sometimes people feel like talking more just when they are about to leave someone." This kind of comment will help the child understand that part of his or her desire to open up to you is related to having to part from you. Later on, after you have seen the child several times, you may want to make a comment about this behavior by saying something like, "Here we are talking and you're telling me a lot of important things that I'm eager to hear more about, but I wonder how come you're telling me about it now? Sometimes people do this just before they're ready to leave, which makes it much harder to leave, because you've got so much to talk about." In general, whatever the child's particular style, you want first to help him or her understand that the end of the interview is coming and then to make the child aware of his or her reaction to the impending separation.

Near the end of the interview, with 5 or 10 minutes remaining, I often ask some structured questions. Usually by that time the child has indicated the nature of the family constellation. If he has not, I might ask him about his family: "Tell me about. . . ." Typically, I will get the first association—"Mommy, oh she's never home." Father—"He makes lots of money." Baby brother—"Takes away my toys." Sometimes you get a startling response. Father—"Oh, he kills people." "Tell me about that." "Oh, I was just kidding."

Often I ask the child if he ever has dreams—daydreams and night dreams—and a very high percentage tell me their dreams. Occasionally one hears an interesting dream that helps to support or refute hypotheses formed in the course of the interview. Depending on the time and on what else I have learned, I might ask a child about school or friends to hear first associations, or I might ask if the child has any questions he wants to ask me. I usually try to include the latter by saying, "You have told me a lot. Is there anything I can tell you?" Very often I get something interesting in response. Let me add, however, that concluding structured questions yield information of less value than what you gathered during the unstructured period of the interview.

The phases of an unstructured interview proceed as follows. In the initial phase the child communicates why she is there, and you clarify and support her feelings. In the middle phase, the child begins to get to know you better and to develop a relationship with you. Here, you observe the child in all the categories as her story unfolds, making helpful comments to further associative trends and synthesizing clarifications. The final phase, signifying "good-bye," shows how the child deals with separation. At this time, you may also wish to ask a few structured questions.

CASE ILLUSTRATIONS OF THE TECHNIQUE OF CONDUCTING AN UNSTRUCTURED INTERVIEW

In order to illustrate the principles discussed above, we will now reconsider some thematic aspects of the initial, middle, and final phases of the clinical interviews presented in Chapter 4. It may prove useful to refer back to those interviews cited.

In the initial phase of the interview in Case 1, Doug finally reaches out with his "Hi" after some moments of paralyzing anxiety, then continues without reserve. Displaying some emotional hunger, he talks of his need for security (saving money) and his worries about illness. It is his choice to open the dialogue by letting the interviewer know that he is in distress and willing to reach out. Hints of deeper concerns also emerge as themes of physical damage are elaborated early in the interview, perhaps suggesting what Doug may be afraid of in developing a new relationship.

In the middle part of the interview we see the theme get more organized and the plot thicken. Doug talks about saving his money "to take care of future emergencies," then becomes concerned with "robbers and lazy bums" hurting people, stealing his money, and also perhaps hurting his brother. Here it is not clear who he is referring to as "robbers and lazy bums." Is it a part of him that would like to "rob others" and perhaps "hurt my brother," or is he expressing some potential worries about the interviewer? The interviewer could be the villain who would rob him and harm his brother. Perhaps he is referring to somebody else, or to a mixture of all of the above. In any event, we see conflict arising between his wish to be secure—to save and have plenty of money—and his fear of lazy bums, robbers, and other thieves who could hurt him.

The interviewer then makes a clarifying comment indirectly, by thinking out loud about robbers without trying to lead Doug in any particular direction—such as seeing himself, the interviewer, or family members as the robbers—because on his own Doug is developing this theme and its conflictual sides. Tone of voice shows that the interviewer's clarification is meant only to underline the concern. (Later on, perhaps in the treatment situation, one might make a more explicit clarification as the particular meaning Doug was elaborating became more understandable.)

It is also interesting to note how Doug moved into the last part of the interview. The prospect of separation evokes his underlying emotional hunger: he wants to continue playing games, to take things with him, and to be assured that he will be able to return. We observe that, instead of demonstrating overt anger as do some chil-

dren who have a great deal of emotional hunger, Doug tries to reassure himself by taking a symbol of the interview home with him
as well as by seeking assurances of the continuation of the sessions.

The interview with Joan in Case 3 further illustrates the characteristic progression of the unstructured interview. In the earliest
part of the interview Joan reveals her interest in things sticking out
(the Bobo's nose) and in breaking off what sticks out. Following this
she becomes more structured, thereby perhaps indicating some anxiety about this interest. We might hypothesize that she is opening up
her interview by saying that she herself is anxious about "sticking
her neck out" in terms of what she will relate in this setting and that
she is worried about being "broken off." In other words, she is anxious about what she feels to be her own tendency to open up and let
things stick out. Or perhaps she is conveying the way she relates to
others, that if they offer to get to know her, she is afraid she will
break off what they extend. In the opening phase we may speculate
but cannot know whether she is talking about herself or others or
some combination. We do get a picture of how she perceives the
situation: something is going to begin sticking out and then something
may get broken off.

In the middle of the interview she starts to elaborate a conflict.
She is concerned about the wolf pretending to be grandmother, and
then becomes curious and suspicious about the mirrors on the wall.
The interviewer comments that Little Red Ridinghood must have been
scared and unsure about the world, and that she, Joan, must be
unsure about what's happening in this situation, whether there are
wolves around and what these mirrors mean. As will be recalled,
after a moment of apprehension, after tearing off the paper she was
drawing on, she began a theme with the policeman doll and flirted
with the idea of dropping it out the window. The plot deepened with
the scene of the dolls in the toilet. Through these developments as
well as subsequent ones, Joan showed that she was able to use the
clarification of a possible conflict she was experiencing to elaborate
themes expressing her concerns in an extraordinarily rich and dramatic fashion.

Near the end of the interview Joan talks about a dream in
which witches give out "bread with poison on it"; her father eats this
bread and dies. After relating the dream, Joan puts a block under her
dress, shows concern with the interviewer's note-taking, and relates
how her mother stole "Hanukkah money" from her. There is a quality
of emotional hunger at this point, as though she wants to go on and
on about these various concerns. In response to the impending separation she might be saying, "I have a lot more to tell you about many
scary things," and "I'm not sure how to understand this experience."

Did somebody get poisoned, tricked, or have things stolen from her? I feel uneasy about my own body." Such expressions of fearful uncertainty about what happens in relationships with other people might be echoes of the stick-out–break-off theme heard at the beginning of the interview.

The Case 4 interview with Cathy is also instructive. She begins by setting up a family scene using the toilet as a chair, then says that she has to clean the toilet first. Her opening seems to be one of trying to discover what she may and may not do, or perhaps how much she may or may not regress in the situation. In a sense she is saying, "Hello, how are you. What gives here? Is this a place where I have to be clean or can I be messy?" She gives a hint that this may be a general concern in her life, that this is how she greets a new situation.

This concern continues in a muted way throughout the opening phase as she begins to develop her themes. Later, during the middle phase, when she is playing with the salt and getting it all over everything, she mentions that her mother "wouldn't let me do that." Again perceiving an attitude of "should I or shouldn't I," "can I or can't I," the interviewer comments that Cathy might be concerned with rules, and how they differ between here and home. Cathy then becomes more expansive, sharing her fantasies of being aggressive with mother, although again showing the theme of doing and undoing: "I threw things at mother, no I didn't"; "I kick mother, no I don't." Nevertheless, Cathy shows more freedom after the clarification and eventually comes to the point where she not only talks about her mother and her concerns with bombs, but wants to confide "a secret about Mother throwing a hamburger at Daddy."

As the end of the hour approaches, after relating themes of aggression about monsters and scary doctors and then punching me in the arm, Cathy suddenly becomes very curious. She looks in drawers and pretends no one knows what she is doing, indicating some sneakiness. She says that she has "more stories" in a flirtatious, expansive manner. Thus we see her dealing with separation: continuing the development of her thematic concerns about what is permitted and what is not permitted; giving free vent to her underlying feelings, wishes, and interests; and also saying in effect, "I have much more to offer you." She leaves on a confident note. There is no emotional hunger, no anger, no expression of relief. Rather, a confident statement is made. She conveys that there is more to discover, lots of things and many people she is interested in. She also hints that she has something in her own private "drawers," i.e., her own stories, which leaves the interviewer with a feeling of curiosity.

Readers may find it useful to review the other interviews presented in Chapter 4 or interviews of their own in order to study how the different phases of the clinical interview evolve. By following the basic principles discussed earlier, that is, facilitating communication, tolerating discomfort, and maximizing observations, the diagnostician will be able to gather sufficiently rich data from any type of child. If the diagnostician is unable to observe what a child communicates, that does not mean that the child is in fact uncommunicative. Even the child who sits for 45 minutes and refuses to utter a word tells you something profound. By making use of the observational framework presented in Chapter 2, including observing the presymbolic developmental levels and the presymbolic aspects of each category in the context of the unstructured interview, you will find that it is impossible for a child to be either uninteresting or uninformative.

6

Constructing a Formulation Based on a Developmental Approach

THE CLINICIAN MAKING ASSESSMENTS of children has available, in addition to the diagnostic interviews, various other types of relevant data. The results of psychological testing; the child's developmental history; school reports; consultations; medical and neurological evaluations as needed; sensory, motor, and language studies, if appropriate; assessments of family functioning as a whole as well as of individual family members—all are necessary to the diagnostic process. From the data of clinical interviews alone, however, you can deduce useful hypotheses that may then be refined and further developed in the light of information from the other sources. In this way the systematic observations made in the diagnostic interview can become the cornerstone of your assessment and diagnostic formulation. The question dealt with in this chapter is, What is the best approach to take in considering the observations and impressions gathered in interviewing the child? The approach I advocate here is a developmental one.

Using each of the observational categories we have been discussing—i.e., physical and neurological development, mood, relatedness, affect, use of environment, thematic development, and your own subjective feelings—your judgment about the particular child is made by comparing his or her functioning with the age-appropriate styles and levels of functioning. In other words, after you have compiled detailed descriptions of the child's functioning in each category, ask yourself how this child's capacities compare with the age- and developmental stage–appropriate norms.

Table 3-1 in Chapter 3, which offers illustrative examples of developmental phase- and age-appropriate levels of functioning for each category, will help orient you to these standards. Their usefulness lies in guiding you in the development of your own internal chart so that awareness of these expectations will reside at an intuitive as well as at a cognitive level. The internal chart takes form gradually as you gain experience with scores of clinical interviews. Then you literally feel something amiss when you deal with a child who is not functioning at age-appropriate levels, and this intuitive sense is the clue that prompts a search for what, specifically, the child is doing or saying (or not doing or saying) that falls short of expectations.

A special word about *content* is in order here. Judgments about the content of a child's themes, in contradistinction to those about thematic structural elements such as organization and sequence, should be held in abeyance until you have fully understood the unique circumstances of the child's life. With regard to issues of content, knowledge of the familial, societal, and cultural factors at work will contribute importantly to your interpretation. Thus, you may notice that a child's content seems idiosyncratic and out of sync with what is usually seen at this phase and age. In order to judge whether this child's concerns reflect an extraordinarily adaptive coping strategy, a reasonable manner of coping, or a pathological style, you must first become knowledgeable about the family circumstances and the historical perspective that engendered these concerns. As your experience broadens and deepens, your sense of age-appropriate concerns in varying contexts will sharpen correspondingly and surprises will occur less often.

With respect to those categories that reflect process and structure—e.g., thematic organization, organization of affects, and relatedness (or nonrelatedness)—the experienced clinician finds that the questions and tentative hypotheses generated by the interview hold up fairly well when examined in the light of information from other sources.

Let us say that your internal chart of developmental phase- and age-appropriate levels of functioning is reasonably well developed and you have justifiable confidence in your abilities to observe a child in the interview in all the senses we have previously discussed.

At this point I would suggest to you a framework for forming hypotheses regarding a child's developmental status based on the interview data alone. The framework consists of a series of three basic questions and related subquestions. Using the observations made in each of the categories, you seek a determination, or hypothetical answer, to each question.

The first question in the series is: What is the level of the basic ego functions, including 1) the organic or neurophysiological components of ego functioning and 2) the functional or psychological aspects of ego functioning, and how do these levels compare with the age-appropriate developmental levels?

To determine the level of functioning of the organic components of the ego you would examine such aspects as motor coordination, sensory systems, sensorimotor integration, cognition, language, and the capacity to concentrate and focus attention. Intelligence, a product of multiple factors, would be included in your determination, as would specific cognitive or learning difficulties insofar as they are based on the physical maturation of the central nervous system. Since intelligence and cognitive difficulties are rarely determined solely by "organic" factors, however, you must always consider the functional factors as well.

With regard to psychological aspects of ego functioning, compare the child's actual psychological capacities with the age-expected capacities for reality testing, impulse regulation, mood organization, and stability; also compare the child's capacities to organize and refine a sense of self, to integrate and organize emotions, and to think.

Certain categories are obviously pertinent to the task of assessing ego functions. Data from the second category, relatedness, will help to determine the age-appropriateness of the child's capacity for forming human relationships as well as his or her capacity to delineate a sense of self. Data from the third category, mood, will help to determine if the child is below the age-appropriate level in the capacity to organize and stabilize mood. Your descriptive data in the fourth category will yield clues to whether the basic structure of the child's personality in terms of organizing emotions and integrating them with thought is at the appropriate age level. With regard to the way the child deals with anxiety, look for grossly disorganizing anxiety that is inconsistent with age expectations. For example, we would not be surprised at disorganizing anxiety in a 3-year-old, but would be concerned if the same degree of disorganization appeared after an anxious interaction with a 7- or 8-year-old.

In looking at the thematic category, we would not be as concerned with thematic sequence as with the capacity for age- and phase-appropriate thematic organization. Does an 8-year-old seemingly bring themes "out of left field," as illustrated in Chapter 2 by the child who talked about his body falling apart without any buildup or link to earlier themes, thereby demonstrating a possible difficulty in distinguishing fantasy from reality and/or the beginning of a "thought disorder"? With regard to one's own subjective impressions, at times one will get an uncanny sense of something most unusual about a child, which may be a tip-off that his or her personality organization is not age-appropriate.

Having a developmental map of early ego functions in mind will help in this task. For example, determining how well a child focuses and engages and organizes intentional gestural communication tells you about the presymbolic aspects of relationships, mood, affects, and thematic organization. Observing whether a child uses words or pretend play to represent experience and how he creates logical bridges between his symbolic productions tells you about his representational worlds. The child may be at different levels for different emotional realms.

Once you have compared the child's level of functioning with the age-appropriate norms in our observational categories, you should ask yourself about the "autonomous" ego functions, namely, creativity, curiosity, and intellectual capacity. You want to know if the child has strengths or weaknesses in these areas of ego functioning.

If you do nothing else in a diagnostic session, make sure that you observe whether a child's basic ego functions are below the age-appropriate level. You do not want to overlook the fact that an 8-year-old with superficial learning problems is functioning psychologically at a 5- or 6-year-old level. Such oversights are frequently made with children because of the subtleties associated with the functioning appropriate to each particular age.

With very young children, for example, in whom you expect the distinction between reality and fantasy to be blurred, it is sometimes difficult to determine whether a child is at an age-appropriate level. A 3½-year-old who shows you no evidence of realistic interaction with the environment may be manifesting less than age-appropriate functioning along the lines of differentiating self from nonself. On the other hand, if you notice this lag intermittently in some areas and not in others, you may be witnessing a normal developmental performance. A 4- or 5-year-old child may say he is scared because there is a monster who comes in at night, hides under his bed, and keeps him from sleeping. When you ask if that is a dream, the child says, "No, that's a real monster. I'm afraid to look under my bed." At these early ages the capacity for fantasy is often quite robust. Yet many children, if you press them by saying, "It's make-believe even though I know it feels real," will admit that you have put it correctly.

They can make the distinction with support. On the other hand, you may see children who are unable to make the distinction. In many such cases further inquiry may reveal that their problem in this area is narrowly circumscribed, the boundary between primary- and secondary-process thinking being impaired only in regard to certain kinds of fearful fantasies; you may even uncover structured phobias.

In general, you have to make very subtle distinctions in assessing the basic ego functions of children ages 3 to 6, for these are the years when such ego functions are actually developing. Your picture of whether basic functions—such as differentiation of self from nonself, as well as the capacity to test reality—are below expectations depends largely on issues of context and pervasiveness. If a blur between fantasy and reality occurs in one limited context—for instance, at night, when even adults hearing a noise may think there is an intruder in the house—you would not think of a lag in reality testing. If, however, a 4-year-old thinks "crooks are following me" all day long, you may consider the possibility that there is a distortion in certain age-appropriate ego functions.

Although the difficulty of assessing basic ego functions is greater when you are observing younger children, and thus sometimes the source of inappropriate diagnoses, older children can also be hard to assess. For example, there are latency-age children with organized delusional systems who keep their problems fairly secret. They may give you one or two clues in the playroom—a bizarre stare or a weird giggle—but on the whole behave in a reasonably appropriate manner, causing you to miss their inability to differentiate fantasy from reality.

It may be especially hard to assess basic ego functioning in troubled teenagers. You may see teenagers with multiple symptoms of depression and anxiety and, with so much to assess in terms of symptoms, simply fail to observe more severe psychopathology, such as a basic deficit in ego functioning. Such misses are exceedingly unfortunate because often, if the treatment program is not aimed at the most fundamental problem, a child capable of full recovery and growth is unable to realize it.

For instance, take the case of a young woman with multiple phobias who was seeing a hypnotherapist. Beginning in adolescence, the girl had seen four or five psychiatrists who had focused in various ways on her "neurotic" symptoms. She had always functioned superficially well and had the kind of symptoms that could easily be viewed as neurotic. No one ever saw that there was an underlying difficulty in organizing themes and rich, age-appropriate affects. In other words, there was a subtle thought disorder. By the time she was seeing the hypnotherapist, she had deteriorated to the point of being unable to work or live on her own. Whether this deterioration could have been prevented cannot be determined; yet, from the material presented it appeared that there would have been a good chance of improvement rather than deterioration if her core vulnerability in basic ego functions—rather than merely the more superficial symptoms—had been treated.

In addition to looking for obvious departures from age-appropriate norms of ego functioning—i.e., delusions, hallucinations, loosening of associations in the sense we have talked about, wildly inappropriate affects—it is important to be attuned to the subtler departures: those that give you a sense of a hazy boundary between the self and the nonself. This haziness arises from disordered development in the period from ages 2 to 4, when the capacity for symbol making begins to emerge and the developmental task of differentiating self from other at a symbolic level is achieved.

Some people never quite master the differentiation of self from other at the level of mental representation. Such people will temporarily manifest less than age-appropriate reality testing, affect modulation, and integration of thought and affect, and then quickly recover appropriate age-level behavior. Basically, they suffer an impairment in the capacity to differentiate fully all experiences that are related to the self from all those related to the nonself. To spot such an impairment in the children you interview, look into the categories covering emotional tone and relatedness; particularly examine the child's capacity to organize themes and communication patterns, and be aware of your own subjective feelings.

By conceptualizing the child's functioning in a developmental framework (i.e., comparing the child's functioning levels with age-appropriate levels) one gains a precision of identification not readily available in the pathological descriptive framework. Thus, rather than having a global diagnosis to work with (e.g., the child is psychotic), it is more helpful to a therapist's treatment program to have the specific ego impairments spelled out (e.g., the capacity for thematic organization in this 6-year-old is at the level of a 3-year-old). Identification of the child's problem in a developmental context allows the therapist to see more clearly the degree and area of impairment.

Assuming that you have ascertained that the personality organization (basic ego functioning) is intact, the second question in the series is: What is the degree of ego rigidity in relation to age-appropriate rigidity? Or conversely, is this child capable of phase- and age-appropriate flexibility? Can this child experience the ranges of feelings, thoughts, and interpersonal relationship patterns appropriate to his or her age and developmental phase? Can the child employ the appropriate adaptive, coping, and defensive maneuvers?

Certain children are able to maintain intact personality functioning (reality testing, impulse regulation, mood stabilization, and overall affect organization) only at the expense of relinquishing age- and phase-expected flexibility. Such children may forgo genuine contact with others, for example; their relationships are shallow, mechanical, devoid of the warmth of human intimacy. Others may give up assertiveness or aggressiveness; they are passive, compliant, and mildly withdrawn. In such children we see a "walling off" of certain areas of human experience—pleasure and intimacy in the former; assertiveness and mastery in the latter—in the service of maintaining their capacity for intact personality functioning. These are children who are operating on a narrow stage and playing out but one drama. All their affects are colored by this one drama. They have constricted their range of experiences.

For example, you may interview a child who cannot tolerate any experience of human feelings. He tends to live in an impersonal and concrete experiential world where he relates mainly to inanimate objects. Although such a child might come in and talk to you in a seemingly normal way, you sense his impersonal level of attachment. The child might focus on inanimate objects in the room, show considerable interest in how things work, and be quite organized and logical in approaching the inanimate world, but a spark would be missing; such a child lacks a range of affects and allows no meaningful affective involvement with you or with friends, parents, or siblings. He may talk about building an airplane with friends, but you get no sense either of pleasure or competitive aggressiveness. This boy, early in life and perhaps with good reason, may have made a pivotal, though not intentional, decision; perhaps one could say his developmental processes made a decision for him. He may have decided that in order to protect his basic ego functions, in order to remain in this world and not go "crazy," he has to limit himself to a range of experience that excludes human feelings.

Other examples of less severe constriction include children who, for fear of losing mother's love, may give up any awareness of angry feelings, and experience only sadness and depression. In other words, they are frightened because they were never able to work out that they could get angry at mother and that she would not abandon them as a result. Their basic ego development has occurred; therefore, their basic reality testing is intact. Because they are frightened of the conscious experience of anger and of the behavioral experience of assertiveness, however, the whole area of anger and assertiveness is cut off.

Often children with some degree of ego rigidity do not have problems until much later in their lives when one or another developmental demand puts them under stress. An illustration would be the person who had peer relationships on a fairly concrete level as a child but felt extremely uncomfortable when it came time to date and have more intimate relationships. Only then, in adolescence, did he begin to feel isolated and to experience depression. On reflection, you would be able to see a pattern stemming from childhood in which certain kinds of pleasurable and affectionate yearnings were walled off.

Another example would be the child who throughout her early development demonstrated a strong and assertive character. As she matured, she took over many leadership roles and was considered a healthy, model teenager. Yet, as she entered her twenties and separated from her family, she became quite depressed and withdrawn. What had been overlooked in her youth was her inability to deal with passivity and its associated longings. Early in life she had walled off affects and themes related to passivity. A playroom session with such a person at the age of 8 might have revealed an absence of empathy, dependent yearnings, an inability to cope with loss and to experience sadness, and an overinvestment in assertive and aggressive themes. If the situation had been reversed, that is, if she had been a passive, preoccupied child who was not doing well in school, she might well have come to the attention of a teacher and received necessary treatment.

As indicated, both intuitive awareness and cognitive knowledge of age-appropriate proclivities are crucial for assessing ego rigidity. Use the information from the descriptive categories to make this assessment of a specific child. In the category of relatedness (again, assuming you have already determined that there is a capacity for relatedness), look at the style and range in terms of the age expectations. Does this 5-year-old, who ought to be capable of a rich wide-ranging emotional style, actually have a shallow and constricted style? Is this 8-year-old, who should be capable of some empathy, sharing, and mutual regard, clinging and demanding? In the category of mood, is there a fixed stereotypical mood inconsistent with age-appropriate capacities? Is the 5-year-old—who ought to be expansive and joyous—sad, depressed, and sober-looking during the entire interview? Is the range of affect in an 8-year-old limited to competitive strivings with games of shooting and one person beating up another, or is there a range of affects reflecting competitiveness, lovingness, protectiveness, and orderliness? In the category of thematic development, look at the richness and depth of themes elaborated. Are certain age-appropriate themes absent? For instance, take the case of a 5-year-old who is not developing intricate family dramas involving competition, rivalry, intrigue, and curiosity but instead is playing out only one drama reflecting emotional hunger and the fear of being hurt. The richness and depth of the themes clue you to those areas that are being experienced and those that are not.

The child's affects, thoughts, and interpersonal experience—to the extent that they are revealed in the interview—give you a detailed picture of the relative richness or poverty of the child's inner life, which you can then compare with the expected norm. Moreover, they give you a sense of what it feels like inside the child's skin. For example, a child may not have any overt problems, but the shallowness of his inner life is conveyed by the few primitive affects he manifests. You observe only some sadness, a little envy, a little jealousy; you see no capacity for love, empathy, or sharing; no competitiveness or assertiveness; you sense the child's inner emptiness. You see him play with peers, but in shallow ways. Your notes show that the thematic content in the playroom failed to develop; that your own customary interest, curiosity, and personal warmth failed to materialize. In sum, even though there were no major symptoms in evidence—in fact, it was not even clear why the child was brought in—you have both observed and sensed that he has little depth. What is missing can be assumed to be walled off or rigidified. Something in this child's personality is not being represented, differentiated, integrated, and synthesized.

The concept of rigidity is relative rather than absolute. I like to use the analogy of a balloon to describe this range of internal human experiences. The balloon is fully and evenly inflated in children who are functioning at the age-appropriate level in all facets of the observational categories. In children whose functioning is impaired in a circumscribed area (e.g., a structured phobia), a weak spot or bruise is visible in one area of the balloon, but the balloon is flexible and can stretch to maintain its symmetry. The look of the balloon that represents children with more extensive impairment would be lopsided; some sections are stretched tight while others are limp and collapsed. Such children would be functioning to some degree—able to attend school, for example, and to carry out adequate reality testing—but they have developed pervasive character distortions such as obsessive-compulsive or hysterical patterns. To complete the analogy, balloons of such poor-quality material that they burst at the slightest provocation represent children with the most flagrantly impaired basic ego functioning. These children would be spotted by means of the first question in the series. Unlike children with some degree of flexibility in basic ego functioning, such deeply troubled children are incapable of encapsulating their problems or narrowing their range of experience to protect themselves. Rather, they often exacerbate their difficulties because their reality testing is totally inadequate.

Thus, a child hampered by some age-inappropriate rigidity, finding himself in over his head, will swim back to shore and sit on the beach; but a child whose basic ego functioning is age-inappropriate will, in similar circumstances, swim farther out and deny, often grandiosely, that there is any trouble at all.

To illustrate the difference between a less-than-flexible balloon and one of the poorest quality, let us say you are observing an 8-year-old girl who is facing a stressful situation; you ask yourself, What is her range of coping strategies? For instance, if she has only mild rigidity, she might use a little denial, some reaction formation or projection, or, more sophisticatedly, she might show some capacity for sublimatory channels. With moderate rigidity, she instead would become somewhat irritable, as well as a little negativistic or argumentative, but would remain continually involved with family and friends. A severe impairment would be indicated if she suffered a major regression and withdrew from human relationships; began behaving negativistically and impulsively; began to lose control of urine and feces.

Let us now look at the kinds of behavior that characterize various degrees of rigidity in the functioning of basic ego structures that are fundamentally intact. At the level of serious impairment (the lopsided balloon), you might see paranoia, mild schizoid patterns, or passive-aggressive patterns as a basic way of life. If such behavior patterns are not present, you want to see if only a small part of the balloon is cut off, which would represent a relatively moderate walling off of experience.

An example would be the child who evinces pleasure; who is sweet and somewhat passive; whose range of affects shows no assertiveness, aggression, or competition, but does show all the other age-appropriate affects; and whose thematic content matches the affect—that is, it shows no competitiveness, envy, jealousy, assertiveness, or fighting. Although the child's mood and the basic relatedness to you are appropriate, certain age-appropriate components do not emerge in the course of the interview. Such a configuration of observations is consistent with a child whose flexibility is not at the appropriate age level. Such a child is more psychologically developed than a schizoid child who gives up all affective involvement, for the former gives up only the affects that scare him or her. The former child has not experienced a major "shutdown," or cutting off of experience early in life, but instead has experienced certain affects as frightening and has therefore decided to give them up. The fact that the child has had some involvement—albeit brief—with the now missing pieces of his experiential world will make your therapeutic task easier.

The mildest manifestation of rigidity (an abscess in the balloon) could be termed an encapsulated limitation. Here, the overall ego structure is basically flexible in all of the categories mentioned. By and large, the child is able to engage the world in an age-appropriate manner. That is to say, the child's neurophysiology, human relationships, moods, range of affects and stability of affects under stress, and thematic organization (particularly the sequence of themes) are all age-appropriate. However, there is a contextually significant area that is walled off; often you will find it to be closely associated with any symptoms that the child may be suffering. In certain areas where there are conflicts, neurotic mechanisms work to encircle the conflicts and keep them from spreading, and thus protect the child from regressing characterologically. Using our analogy of a theater stage, the stage of a child with encapsulated limitations is the appropriate size, and sound enough to contain wide-ranging dramas that have both age-appropriate themes and themes from earlier phases of development. But you notice some bumps and snags in the flooring, which the child has to avoid as he or she performs the drama.

An encapsulated disorder—e.g., a phobia such as fear of elevators—protects the flexibility of the rest of the personality in the same way an abscess protects the rest of the body from infection. Let us say that a child is referred to you because of marked symptoms of a phobic nature. The child is doing well in school and enjoying good peer relationships; he develops themes around competition, aggression, and envy as well as compassion, empathy, loving, and caring. You feel he has handled his range of concerns in an organized way. But as you look closely at the thematic sequence, which is where you get your clues to what is going on with such a child, you see that, in addition to the symptoms of nightmares, phobia, or mild sibling rivalry, there are related problems. You observe an undue amount of anxiety around certain themes. For instance, there is a sudden disruption when the subject of competition with siblings arises. In response to your comment, "I know kids have a lot of different feelings about brothers and sisters," the child, instead of opening up this area, shows some constriction. He says, "Oh, yes. Of course, most kids love their brothers and sisters and they ought to," and continues to talk about the protective, loving dimensions of having siblings while strictly avoiding competitive, angry thoughts. Even more commonly, a child with a flexible ego structure who has some Oedipal conflicts may talk a lot about the competition and anger but say nothing about his curiosity concerning the more pleasurable interests that arise in the context of the family drama. Such interests have been walled off. As you move in on this and say, "You know, kids usually have a lot of curiosity and interest about what goes on with their parents," the child says, "Oh no, not me," or "That doesn't happen," or "I don't know what you are talking about," suddenly becoming naive and acting "dumb" when you touch on this anxiety-laden theme. Here you see a walling off of the experiential world in a contextually narrow range and area, often dynamically defined. If you were to ask a healthy Oedipal child the same question, he might talk about how he tried to break into the parents' bedroom, or how he went into the bathroom with his father.

An encapsulated limitation in flexibility such as a phobia might seem more serious than a moderate but pervasive constriction because the former is more obvious. A phobia in an otherwise flexible ego structure can be seen as a developmental accomplishment, however, in the sense that the capacity for neurosis implies a high level of integration in a rather flexible ego structure. Nagera (1966) has discussed the notion that the infantile neurosis, which forms the foundation for later neurotic conflicts, reflects a substantial developmental achievement. That is, a child cannot be only neurotic until he or she has achieved an Oedipal—and therefore rather advanced—level of development. Thus, a neurotic disorder in itself implies that development has proceeded well in terms of personality flexibility.

It should be emphasized, however, that an encapsulated limitation is one that successfully protects the personality's flexibility. If the symptom in question does interfere with going to school, having friends, or enjoying the full range of pleasurable and assertive affects and themes, then we are not dealing with an encapsulated limitation, which we have defined as one that protects the personality. The behavior of a child with an encapsulated limitation is not seriously below the appropriate age level. Of course, neurotic conflicts can and do occur in the presence of other, more pervasive impairments. You must make your diagnosis systematically. If the child's developmental level in certain ego functions is significantly below normal, that is your primary diagnosis. You must patch up the cracks in the stage before you can work on the dynamics of a particular neurotic conflict.

From a developmental perspective, a pure encapsulated disorder would suggest only circumscribed difficulties at the stage of representational differentiation. Character constriction would suggest difficulties at the stages of representational elaboration and differentiation. Severe personality disorders and borderline states would suggest contributions from prerepresentational levels, as would the more severe disorders. For these types of difficulties, the basic capacity for prerepresentational differentiation (i.e., behavioral reality testing) is often compromised, as is the stability of the capacity to engage with and be related to others.

Each level of inflexibility (constriction) may be further delineated in terms of specific subtypes. In other words, a limitation in the flexibility of the balloon can take many different forms, which are discussed below.

MAJOR CONSTRICTIONS

The integrity of basic personality functioning may be maintained at the price of flexibility in the overall character structure. Massive avoidance of dangerous areas of life experience, or massive inhibition of wishes, thoughts, or affects, allows the child to stay away from situations that will cause a breakdown of ego functions (e.g., severe schizoid or paranoid characters, negativistic personalities, severe depressive characters, or narcissistic disorders).

Children with such a constricted adjustment do not normally show signs of ego defects. They function adequately—within the constrictions of their characters—without special vulnerability to fragmentation. The price they pay is a serious restriction of their life experiences. Such a child may live a relatively symptom-free life by avoiding stressful experiences. For example, a child with a limitation in the capacity to modulate affect might use avoidance to stay away from feeling states that are perceived as dangerous. In the clinical interview one might notice a highly idiosyncratic or *very* restricted thematic and affective range as well as style of relatedness. Specific subtypes of constrictions and impairments in flexibility are outlined below.

One major constriction is *limitation of experience of feelings and/ or thoughts*. For example, a child does not experience warm, loving feelings and avoids intimate one-to-one relationships (e.g., the schizoid type of personality). He may appear distant and aloof in interviews, remaining on an emotionally flat level in spite of significant time spent with the interviewer. Another child (e.g., one who is chronically depressed) restricts her internal affective experience; she does not permit herself angry or assertive feelings, but experiences only passive sadness. Behaviorally she is limited to apathetic, mildly withdrawn actions. Yet another child may not be able to tolerate dependent wishes, and will appear too self-reliant and somewhat unconcerned.

Another constriction is *alteration and limitation of pleasure orientation*, as, for example, manifested in the perversions. This loss of flexibility is often accompanied by a stereotyped, intense pleasure orientation limited to a few areas. That is, certain kinds of pleasure cannot be experienced. In the interview, the style of relatedness, affects, and thematic sequence may have a persistent tone centering on one theme, such as sadistic pleasure or a particular body part, without any signs of compassionate, warm, empathic pleasure. The behavior may also express sadistic themes and concerns with certain anatomical zones.

Major externalization of internal events, such as conflicts, feelings, and thoughts, is another character distortion. The child who externalizes hostile internal wishes or feelings may perceive aggression as persistently coming from the outside. Themes of "they are out to get me" may dominate the interview. Another, less severe syndrome of externalization is seen in those children who externalize perceptions about themselves (such as low self-esteem) onto others (e.g., saying in the interview, "I know you find me icky"); or those who act out their internal conflicts by polarizing their views, taking one side of the conflict themselves and provoking others to speak for the opposite side. For example, a child might externalize his self-criticism by acting in a way that provokes his parents to be critical of him; or in the interview, by provoking the clinician to manifest a critical attitude.

Another constriction is the *limitation of internalizations necessary for regulation of impulses, affects, and thoughts*. The person with an underlying difficulty in internal regulation does not see his impulsiveness as a symptom. It would, however, become apparent in the interviews; for example, when a theme of separation is immediately followed by a theme of impulsiveness or by impulsive behavior. In the process of the clinical interview such a youngster may demonstrate little patience, continually vacillating between self-gratification ("Where is the candy?") and impulsive behavior (e.g., breaking your furniture).

The child with a *limitation in self-esteem maintenance* manages to maintain surprisingly stable personality superficially (albeit with intolerance for failure and problems with empathy and intimacy). Such children may present a shallow quality of engagement while attempting to impress the interviewer with their own importance. In the interview, they may show little capacity for genuine warmth or empathy and, after a few interviews, will vacillate between relying on the interviewer for a sense of self-worth or self-esteem, and turning to unrealistic grandiose fantasies for such support. If the interviewer is able to engage such children, they may eventually communicate a deep sense of emptiness and vulnerability, with tremendous fear of loss. Such children are constricted in the capacity to experience self-worth, self-esteem, and a range of compassionate and empathic feelings toward others.

Persons with a mild *instability in self-object differentiation* are vulnerable to a limited breakdown of that capacity, followed by reorganization. For example, under stress these children may either lose some control over affect or impulses, or show a disorganization in their thematic sequence. Their lives are not generally unstable because they restrict their experiences to avoid stress, but they can regress toward dedifferentiation. Such children may, therefore, when pressed in an interview, present mild fragmentation in their communication patterns.

MODERATE CHARACTER OR PERSONALITY CONSTRICTIONS

Disorders consisting of moderate character constrictions (e.g., moderate obsessive-compulsive or hysterical personality patterns, some limited impulsive behavior, a tendency toward externalization) involve the same categories of inflexibility of personality (characterological constriction) as above, but to a lesser degree. Only certain aspects of the personality evidence chronic repetitive limitations—in contrast to constriction of the entire personality in more severe disorders.

ENCAPSULATED DISORDERS

Encapsulated disorders protect the flexibility of the personality by producing limited impairments related to symptoms and contextually specific character traits. They differ from characterological constrictions in a very important way; that is, they do not involve avoidance of broad areas of experience. Encapsulated disorders also do *not* involve chronic, repetitive avoidance or limitations of thoughts, wishes, and affects. For example, whereas anger in general is avoided in a character constriction, in an encapsulated disorder only anger directed at a *contextually significant* other might be avoided (e.g., anger at an authority figure associated with one's father). Similarly, a pleasurable feeling will be avoided only in contextually relevant situations. While these feelings are usually identified by dynamic hypotheses, they are also directly observable.

Encapsulated Symptom Disorders

The major limitations and alterations seen in symptom encapsulations are in thought and affect. The first type, *limitation of thought*, is found, for example, in "hysterical" symptoms such as periodic dizziness. Aside from such symptoms the child may function at an age-appropriate level: engage in warm, loving relationships; be assertive; and experience empathy and concern as well as anger and aggression. Only a narrow content area of psychic life dealing with specific wishes (e.g., of a pleasurable nature) is walled off. In the interview, the limitation of thought may become apparent only by the continued absence of this specific content in an otherwise flexible child who evinces a wide range of themes.

The second major type of symptom-encapsulated disorder is *limitation or alteration of affect* (e.g., as seen in obsessive or compulsive patterns). In the interview such children may evince the absence of specific affects in certain contextual situations (e.g., they may not evince anger at the interviewer when such a response would be expected, and/or be unable to evidence thematic trends dealing with anger toward certain contextually significant figures).

Encapsulated disorders are usually not difficult to diagnose. The child shows a broad range of age-appropriate themes and affects, and a reasonable interpersonal engagement with the interviewer. However, in certain contextually evident areas he is capable of only limited affective range and/or thematic depth. There is an obvious disparity between the otherwise flexible personality and the encapsulated areas.

Encapsulated Character Limitations

These disorders present themselves not so much in specific symptoms (phobias, compulsive rituals, or conversion reactions), but rather as subtle limitations in the flexibility of the personality. These disorders differ from the earlier, more severe constrictions of personality both in the narrowness of the area that is limited and in the mildness of the symptoms, if there are any. These disorders are related both to contextually relevant thoughts and affects (e.g., problems with certain types of peers or teachers) and to stress.

They differ from the symptom disorders in that they are not as narrowly focused and often not as intense. An issue may express itself in these disorders in a more diffuse way through a large number of behaviors or thematic expressions. For example, a child with an encapsulated compulsive symptom may repetitively wash her hands; in contrast, a child with an obsessional encapsulated character limitation might be too thorough in his attitude toward school and "getting things completed," may have difficulties expressing his feelings, and may be too self-critical.

A phobic encapsulated symptom (e.g., a fear of height) would be fixed and relatively intense. On the other hand, a phobic encapsulated *character disorder* would probably include phobic attitudes of a milder nature (e.g., a child who is generally fearful and tends to use avoidance a great deal).

In general, neurotic encapsulated character formations may be categorized along the same lines as the more severe character constrictions (with the understanding that the encapsulated disorders are less intense and are related to specific contextually significant experiences rather than to pervasive domains of experience). Thus an *encapsulated limitation of feeling or thought* in a major life area is represented in the child who invariably shies away from the slightest emotional confrontation with authority figures, but whose other areas of emotional experience are not constricted. An *encapsulated alteration in pleasure orientation* might be shown by the child who has difficulty enjoying certain (but not all) types of age-appropriate pleasurable play. An *encapsulated externalization of internal conflict* is seen in the child who blames others for her own behavior in contextually relevant areas. An *encapsulated impairment in self-esteem regulation* is seen in the otherwise emotionally healthy child who easily becomes morose when he loses a game with a contextually significant peer or adult.

TRANSIENT DEVELOPMENTAL CONFLICTS AND STRESSES

To continue the balloon analogy, children with perfectly inflated balloons are fully engaged in a flexible way in phase-appropriate experiences (intrapsychic, interpersonal, etc.). Nevertheless, such children may have transient developmental conflicts; e.g., the child who has nightmares while working through the final stages of the Oedipal phase of development. In addition, one might also observe situational reactions, such as transient anxiety or depression in response to a family crisis. The point is that a healthy, happy child fully involved in age- and phase-appropriate experiences may yet suffer considerable transient discomfort and even symptomatic behavior in the service of developmental progress and adaptive coping with environmental or intrapsychic stress.

Our first two questions—what is the level of basic ego functions, and what is the degree of ego rigidity—tell us about the stage on which the drama is being played, or, in other words, about the structure of the personality. We want to know whether this stage is constructed to meet the age-appropriate standards of integrity and flexibility. If the integrity or flexibility is below expectation, we want to know what parts of the stage are affected and to what degree. If the child is functioning only slightly below age expectations, such a lag might reflect a somewhat slow maturation or the interference of environmental circumstances. But what if the child is clearly one or two major developmental steps behind the age-appropriate level of accomplishment?

Clinical judgments begin to emerge as we compare our observations of the child's functioning with the age-appropriate level. If we have observed that the basic ego functioning is two or three developmental steps below the age-appropriate level—which raises serious questions about the integrity of the personality—then there is a need for further documentation, and the prospect of intensive treatment is considered. Or we may have a child whose basic ego functions are at the age-appropriate level but whose flexibility of personality structure is below expectations by two or three developmental steps. We see that major areas of age-appropriate life experience—such as the capacity for pleasure with peers or the mastery of school requirements—are walled off. In such cases, different considerations regarding treatment recommendations will be required. Another child may show age-inappropriate rigidity in a few confined areas of functioning but otherwise function at age level, indicating many strengths in his personality structure. One sort of treatment recommendation would be made if we judged the disorder to be an encapsulated limitation. If, however, we judge that the area of rigidity is a full developmental level behind age expectations and, moreover, seems fixed there (i.e., if we find no reason to assume that the rigidity is a response to chronic or acute environmental stress), then we would consider different, perhaps more intensive, treatment recommendations aimed at helping the child attain the expected age level in all sectors of development.

This brings us to the third and last question in the series: What are the particular concerns of the child? We look at these concerns in relation to what brought the child in for consultation and in the context of the overall personality structure. In other words, we cannot adequately consider the drama without knowing all about the stage. The drama of aggression, rivalry, and retaliation plays very differently if enacted on a stage that has great holes and cracks versus a stage that is broad, strong, and sturdy. The soundly built stage can well accommodate an intense drama; the poorly made one might very well cave in under the action. All too often, those conducting clinical interviews erroneously zoom in on this third question—the concerns and conflicts—before they make their hypotheses about the integrity of the overall personality structure and its relative flexibility or rigidity.

The child's concerns can be examined from the point of view of their organization, nature, and age appropriateness. The observational categories are helpful to this task. Within the categories, focus more on content than you have done heretofore. Look at the content of the style of relatedness; the particular content and dimensions of the child's mood; the content and sequence of the child's specific predominant affects. Look at the sequence of themes that the child expresses during the interview. Match up the way the child shifts both his relatedness to you and his affects with the sequence of his themes; this matching will help you sketch out the child's particular drama and concerns. As an example, recall the child discussed in Chapter 2, who came in with themes about shooting, shifted to the theme of protecting his brother, and then expressed curiosity about his parents and about his own body. The range of his affects and moods coupled with his specific thematic sequence gave us a picture of some of his particular concerns.

The following outline provides a summary of the categories that are important in determining answers to each of the three questions.

OBSERVATIONAL CATEGORIES FOR CONSTRUCTING A DEVELOPMENTAL DIAGNOSTIC FORMULATION

I. The level of basic ego functions
   A. Organic functioning
      1. Physical and neurological development
   B. Psychological functioning
      1. Capacity for relatedness
      2. Capacity for organizing mood
      3. Capacity for affects and anxieties
      4. Capacity for organizing themes
      5. Subjective reaction of interviewer
      6. Developmental level of 1 to 4 in terms of:
         a) Attention and engagement
         b) Intentional gestural communication
         c) Representational elaboration (sharing meanings)
         d) Representational differentiation (categorizing meanings)
II. The degree of personality rigidity
   A. Style and range of relatedness
   B. Stereotypical mood
   C. Range of affect
   D. Richness and depth of themes
   E. Subjective reaction of interviewer
III. The child's concerns and conflicts
   A. Content and style of relatedness
   B. Content of mood

C. Content and sequence of specific affects
D. Sequence of themes

This chapter has focused on what I have called the developmental approach to diagnosis, and little has been said about the implications for treatment recommendations per se. While treatment will not be considered in this work, a few brief illustrative comments about treatment may be useful and may suggest areas for further discussion. For example, where there are serious developmental lags in basic personality functions (e.g., reality testing, impulse regulations), an intensive program integrating structured supports, such as a therapeutic day program or school and supportive, dynamically oriented psychotherapy, is indicated. As treatment progresses, the supportive and structured features of treatment may in balance give way to a more in-depth approach.

Where there are major rigidities in important sectors of experience (e.g., a child who is one or two developmental stages behind), an intensive, long-term, dynamically oriented psychotherapeutic approach is indicated. The child with more circumscribed but chronic and intense difficulties (e.g., around assertive and aggressive feelings, or around intimate feelings) may also benefit from an intensive approach. In such cases one might expect positive, far-reaching results in a shorter time than with the more major rigidities. In some such cases, where there is a circumscribed difficulty of short duration, short-term dynamically oriented consultations or simply advice to parents, teachers, and others in the child's environment may be enough to help him work out his difficulty.

Finally, where we see a child who is basically at age level in the integrity of basic personality functions and overall flexibility but who is playing out a drama involving conflict, anxiety, and/or depression and is suffering some personal distress, we might consider different approaches. When the distressed child is the most available member of the family, short-term dynamic treatment may be extremely helpful. Where situational circumstances (e.g., a family conflict or school conflict) are contributing, some work with the environment might be indicated. It should be highlighted that work with the environment—family, parents, school, etc.—is usually indicated for all levels of impairment when it is thought that the environment may be harnessed to facilitate development. Furthermore, remedial education and physical-neurological approaches must also be considered where there are even questions of severe lags in central nervous system maturation and/or learning capacities.

A thorough diagnostic workup not only contributes to the overall treatment recommendation but also orients the clinician to the major issues that may need to be taken up in treatment: correcting defects, increasing age-appropriate flexibility, facilitating resolution of age-appropriate conflicts or stresses, etc. While the clinician is always alert to the patient's conflicts, the level and flexibility of ego structure guide the approach.

In this chapter I have tried to show how a particular clinical interview approach lends itself to the formulation of diagnostic hypotheses and preliminary judgments based on developmental considerations. A few comments should be made about the relationship of this approach to the traditional DSM-III-R psychiatric approach to children. As we have seen, the clinical judgments that can be deduced from the interviewing approach advanced here refer to the integrity or developmental level of basic ego functioning and flexibility, and the nature of the child's concerns or conflicts. These judgments parallel the traditional categories of psychiatric disability: psychosis (age-inappropriate level of basic ego functioning); character disorders (major limitations in flexibility in critical sectors of the personality); neurotic disturbances (encapsulated limitations in flexibility around certain areas of experience); and developmental conflicts (the difficulties experienced by the child with the "perfectly inflated balloon" as he or she works through particular developmental tasks). The focus on selected disorders such as depression does not compete with the developmental approach presented here. In fact, the developmental approach helps the clinician determine just what type of depression a child might be evidencing. Is the child having difficulty with regulating mood to such a degree that basic personality functions such as reality testing are interfered with? Or is the child experiencing depressive thoughts in an age-appropriate personality structure?

In addition, a variety of learning and behavioral disorders based on neurological and/or physiological malfunction can be understood in the context of our approach to specific ego functions. These types of disorders, however, are also connected with the psychological aspects of ego functioning. For example, less than full attainment of an expected developmental level may show itself in a global impairment in the capacity to focus concentration; a very circumscribed defect in an ego function, however, may result in only a mild impairment in the same capacity.

Considering the current preference for phenomenology, in contrast to what have been termed "inferred" dynamic states, it is also of interest that our diagnostic approach, although based on dynamic concepts, does not require "a belief" in internal states. Even when referring to children with encapsulated neurotic disorders— those who cannot process experience in a specified narrow domain— you can document the diagnosis *phenomenologically* in your playroom or on psychological testing, just as you can document phenomenologically that a person has hallucinations and delusions. The former is simply a subtler observation requiring, as it were, the high-power lens of your microscope.

For example, observing if a child can represent, through pretend play or with words, concerns with dependency and assertiveness allows you to compare him to another child (without symptoms) who nonetheless shows no evidence of symbolizing a range of emotional patterns and instead either simply behaves out his concerns or quietly inhibits them. The second asymptomatic child may appear healthy, but if he is observed developmentally, we would see limitations. The framework discussed in Chapters 2 and 3 can be used for these observations.

As noted, the clinical judgments that can be derived from our approach are easily translated into the traditional or classical psychiatric concepts. What is being emphasized here, however, is that there may be an advantage to using a developmental framework because its concepts are not limited in explanatory value; they do have implications for pathogenesis and treatment of disorders. The developmental approach suggested here has, in addition, implications for both level of adaptation and level of psychopathology or limitation. Moreover, it has the unique virtue of enabling the interviewer to intuit the way a child experiences his own strengths and weaknesses, and thus to plan appropriate psychotherapeutic approaches.

In practice, the developmental approach presented here may be used together with traditional diagnostic classification schemes. A three-column approach may be used, with diagnoses based on symptoms and personality traits in one column; etiologically based diagnoses in another; and the developmental approach to diagnosis in still another. The developmental approach as described here suggests how the person "organizes" his experience and is in a sense the connection or "experiential pathway" between etiological circumstances and various manifest symptoms. See Table 6-1 for a summary of the developmental categories using the three-column approach. Note that symptom-oriented and etiologically based diagnoses are listed only for illustrative purposes and do not represent the full range of disorders that would correspond to each developmental impairment.

In conclusion, it should be remembered that our discussion has concentrated on the clinical interview with the child and the resultant clinical judgments we can make about the child's functioning. We have not considered a number of the factors—earlier life experiences, current environmental stresses, family communication patterns, and a variety of other biological and environmental factors— that contribute so importantly to the child's functional status. Many would advocate that a full diagnostic system for children should delineate not only the child's manner of organizing his experiential

Table 6-1.   A developmental approach to diagnosis

Illustrative etiologically based diagnoses	Diagnostic categories from a developmental approach	Illustrative diagnoses based on symptoms and personality traits (traditional DSM-III-R, Axes I and II)
	I. Significantly below age-appropriate level of ego functioning (ego defects)	
Infectious encephalopathy. Substance-induced organic mental disorders	A. Basic physical organic integrity of mental apparatus (perception, integration, motor, memory, regulation, judgment, etc.)	Mental retardation Attentional deficit Specific developmental disorders
	B. Structural psychological defects	Pervasive developmental disorder
	1. Thought, reality, testing, and organization	Thought disorders
	2. Perception and regulation of affects	Affective disorders
	3. Integration of affect and thought	
	4. Defect in integration and organization, and/or in differentiation of self- and object-representations	Borderline syndromes
	II. Severe constrictions and alterations in age-appropriate level of ego structure	Behavior disorders Conduct disorders Personality disorders Schizoid disorders
	A. Limitation of experience of feelings and/or thoughts in major life areas (love, learning, play)	
	B. Alterations and limitations in pleasure orientation	Psychosexual disorders
	C. Major externalizations of internal events (e.g., conflicts, feelings, thoughts)	Paranoid personality disorders
	D. Limitations in internalizations necessary for reg-	Impulse disorders

continued

Table 6-1   (continued)

Illustrative etiologically based diagnoses	Diagnostic categories from a developmental approach	Illustrative diagnoses based on symptoms and personality traits (traditional DSM-III-R, Axes I and II)
	ulation of impulses, affect (mood), and thought	
	E. Impairments in self-esteem regulation	Narcissistic disorders
	F. Limited tendencies toward fragmentation of self-object differentiation	Dissociative disorders
	III. Moderate constrictions and alterations in age-appropriate level of ego structure (same as above)	
	IV. Age-appropriate functioning, but with encapsulated disorders	
	A. Neurotic symptom formations	Anxiety disorders
	1. Limitations and alterations in experience of areas of thought (hysterical repression); phobic displacements	Phobic disorders
	2. Limitation and alterations in experience of affects and feelings (e.g., obsessional isolation—depressive turning of feelings against self)	Obsessive-compulsive patterns
	B. Age-appropriate level of functioning, but with neurotic encapsulated character formation	Mild forms of personality disorders
	1. Encapsulated limitation of experience of feelings and thoughts in major life areas (love, work, play)	Mild obsessive-compulsive personality disorders
	2. Encapsulated alterations and limitations in pleasure orientation	Mild psychosexual disorders

Table 6-1   (continued)

Illustrative etiologically based diagnoses	Diagnostic categories from a developmental approach	Illustrative diagnoses based on symptoms and personality traits (traditional DSM-III-R, Axes I and II)
	3. Encapsulated major externalizations of internal events (e.g., conflicts, feelings, thoughts)	Mild paranoid trends
	4. Encapsulated limitations in internalizations necessary for regulation of impulses, affect (mood), and thought	Mild impulse disorders
	5. Encapsulated impairments in self-esteem regulation	Mild narcissistic disorders
	V. Basically age-appropriate, intact, flexible ego structures	
	A. With phase-specific, developmental conflicts	
	B. With phase-specific, developmentally expected patterns of adaptation, including adaptive regressions	Adjustment disorders
	C. Intact, flexible, developmentally appropriate ego structure	

Note.   All of the above structural alterations may have concomitant behavioral alterations, which will usually be described by the symptom cluster diagnoses.

world, which we are focusing on here, but also the dimensions and dynamics of the child's external world, particularly his family environment. I could not agree more with this position and again want to emphasize the limited applicability of this work, which focuses on the clinical interview with the child and is limited in scope to understanding how the child organizes his experiences in this situation.

In the remainder of this chapter I will focus on formulating hypotheses for the clinical interviews presented in Chapter 4, with the aim of illustrating the principles described above and providing important illustrative data on determining the child's concerns or conflicts.

FORMULATIONS FOR CASE 1

The basic organic components of Doug's ego appeared to be intact and at the age-appropriate level, as evidenced by his physical and neurological status (e.g., gross and fine motor coordination, speech, memory, level of intelligence). In contrast, although some basic ego functions were at the age-appropriate level, others were significantly below expectations. Thus, there was a capacity for intense relatedness but it had a hungry quality, indicating a degree of affect hunger more appropriate for a 2- or 3-year-old with some earlier deprivation. Similarly, mood was stable but overall had a depressed quality. The range of affect was not age-appropriate in that it was limited to concerns with illness, danger, robbers, and death. In addition, a quality of affect hunger predominated. On the other hand, Doug's organization and integration of affect and thought were at the age-appropriate level.

Developmentally, he seemed to have partially mastered the early stages of engagement and attention, two-way gestural communication, and early representational elaboration, but with constrictions in range and stability. The stage of representational differentiation evidenced constrictions and vulnerability.

There was some indication of disruptive anxiety around the theme of his father's illness, and there was evidence of thought processes not in accord with a reality orientation when he talked about the "tape recorder" and his brother overhearing us. His thematic organization was therefore significantly below the age-appropriate level, reflecting *not* the organization of a late-latency child but rather the occasional fragmentation (infusion of fantasy into reality) of a 3½- to 4½-year-old. Because Doug showed good capacity to recover a reality orientation, however, there is some question about the degree of the instability (under stress) of his reality orientation and capacity for thematic organization. On the whole, my observations raise a question about the integrity and age-appropriateness of basic ego functions.

While there is evidence of a subtle impairment in basic ego functioning, it should also be noted that for the most part this weakness is protected by a great deal of rigidity in his personality structure. The narrow range of his relatedness (hungry quality), his depressed mood, the narrow range of his affects, and his restricted thematic concerns all point to a rigid, vulnerable personality structure.

The nature of Doug's concerns—as evinced by the content of his relatedness and mood, and the sequence of his affects and themes—points to an unresolved preoccupation with early developmental issues of primitive envy (brother); fear of illness, injury, and death; and an inability to integrate (i.e., some ego splitting) the "robber" in him with his rigid ethical standards and desire to "protect" everyone. The use of projection around the theme of aggression and "being tape-recorded" indicates how disruptive his aggressive feelings are and how fragile are his defenses.

In sum, we have a primitive drama being played out on a very constricted stage with a subtle crack in it. Yet Doug also has a great deal of strength, as evinced by his capacity to relate, his desire for intimacy, his capacity to manifest anxiety and discomfort, and his intelligence.

FORMULATIONS FOR CASE 2

There is some question about the physical and organic aspects of Harold's basic ego functioning. His capacity for concentration seemed significantly below the age-appropriate level as he flitted around in a frenzied way from one activity to the next, at times quite careless about where he was throwing his ball. Many 3½-year-olds, and even some 2½-year-olds, are capable of more focused concentration than this child. By the time a child is 6 to 7½, one expects a more controlled capacity for focused concentration than Harold showed. In addition, his difficulty with "closing his verbal and gestural circles"(i.e., tuning me out) raises the question: Why? Does he have an auditory/verbal processing lag or difficulty, or is he just preoccupied with intense thoughts and feelings? Is he simply easily distracted, or does he evidence a little bit of all of the above?

In terms of the basic functional aspects of his ego, he seemed to be in accord with the reality of the playroom and was able to organize his affects and themes. At the same time, his behavior had a frantic, frenzied quality. He did not disorganize, however, and one theme followed the next in a seemingly logical manner. Moreover, affects and themes were integrated. Also, he did establish a sense of relatedness to me, though it was somewhat fugitive and not as involving as one would hope for a 7½-year-old.

While he came near to hitting me with the ball a few times, he did not show a gross impairment of age-expected impulse control; in addition, later in the interview he was able to respond to limits that I set when he was pulling at the strings of the drapes. Thus, although the basic ego functions were largely intact, he was below age-appropriate functioning in the quality and depth of his relatedness, and in his impulse control, which was not as well integrated as one would hope. With reference to the hypothesis raised above about the age-appropriateness of the organic component of his ego, it is reasonable to ask whether this possible impairment is interfering with and undermining his overall capacity to use intact but slightly below age-appropriate ego functions.

Major limitations in the flexibility of his ego structure were observed. The sequences of his specific affects and themes pointed to his predominant concerns—aggression, power, winning and losing, being Superman, and being fearful of attack. As we saw, there was little affective and thematic development of the empathic, loving, curious dimension of his personality; nor were his concerns with passivity and dependency elaborated. Such marked constrictions are representative of affects and concerns of a younger child.

Constrictions were also noted in the style of his relatedness to me. He was not able to interact and communicate in a deep and rich manner, although he was able to relate superficially with constant eye contact. His relatedness to others may very well be compromised by the overall constriction noted above. That is, his concern with winning and losing—with having power and being attacked—dominates his personality at the expense of the capacities for exploration, warmth, empathy, and passive, dependent longings.

Therefore, we have a child struggling with his aggression and (possibly exaggerated) fear of being attacked. The stage on which he acts is constricted. It also has some fine cracks in those areas related to this boy's ability to modulate his concentration, process auditory-verbal information (possibly), and control his activity level as well as to coordinate and integrate his perceptions with his motor activity.

Developmentally, he has reached the stage of representational differentiation, but only partially. He also has a tendency to be fragmented and partially unstable in his capacities for gestural communication and engagement.

One might hypothesize that Harold is doing the best he can, given his inability to handle the driven quality of his activity level. Feeling driven, he organized himself around a "phallic aggressive mode," a developmental stage where his aggressive inclinations would be ascendant; however, he has been unable to go beyond this level of psychological development. The concerns he is playing out on his constricted and structurally compromised stage, therefore, seem to be overdetermined. There may be functional determinants as well as a maturational organic determinant.

When a child's behavior raises a number of hypotheses, especially ones concerning the organic aspects of ego structure (e.g., auditory processing, perceptual-motor capacities), we certainly want to get additional testing that focuses on these dimensions of ego functioning. These tests may include psychological testing, an occupational therapy evaluation or speech pathology workup, and medical and neurological evaluations.

FORMULATIONS FOR CASE 3

Joan's basic organic integrity and basic ego functions were intact. She showed a rich style of relating and age-appropriate mood, range and organization of affects, and thematic organization and concerns (more or less).

With respect to the degree of age-appropriate flexibility of her personality, we would raise some questions. She needed help in getting started; initially she was silent. Although there was some range, her affects were predominantly focused on apprehensive, fearful, and aggressive issues with hints of curiosity but little demonstration of warm curiosity, empathy, or love. Her thematic expression did develop some richness and depth but not a full age-appropriate range; her concerns were focused on things falling off, people being poisoned and tricked, and the like. Mild fear, suspiciousness, teasing, and testing boundaries with her own aggression (e.g., wanting to throw the policeman doll out the window) dominated at the expense of seductiveness, curiosity, compassion, and early latency-level concerns. Therefore, the thematic sequence was more that of a 4½- to 5-year-old than of a 6-year-old.

Developmentally, she has reached the level of representational differentiation, but with some constrictions and some tendencies toward fragmentation (i.e., one little drama after another, rather than tying all the dramas together into a big play).

Thus, we have a child whose age-appropriate ego structure has some limitations in flexibility. Her concerns with earlier-than-expected developmental issues are nevertheless within her current substage of development, although at the earlier end. Using our theatrical analogy, the stage is intact; it has appropriate width in some areas, is restricted in others, and is playing a drama slightly below age expectations but within Joan's overall developmental substage.

FORMULATIONS FOR CASE 4

Cathy's basic organic integrity and basic ego functions were age-appropriate, as indicated by the level, depth, and organization of personal relatedness; the organization, depth, and richness of affects and themes; and the stability of her mood.

Her flexibility of ego structure was, for the most part, at an age-appropriate level in that during her interview she demonstrated a wide-ranging, rich development of age-appropriate relatedness, affects, and themes with no indications of disruptive anxiety or marked limitations of either positive or negative affects and themes. For example, she engaged the interviewer easily and demonstrated initial concern with the limits of the playroom—in a sense asking if she could give in to her instincts—which is very appropriate behavior for late Oedipal to early latency-stage children (i.e., the tension between letting go versus control). She had clearly progressed to a stable level of representational differentiation.

While the concerns with cleanliness versus messing with the salt indicated some conflict, she was able to elaborate these concerns and use them as a takeoff for an ever-deepening series of communications that touched on themes of exploration, competition (with mother), anger (at brother), and feelings of loss and separation. Near the end of the interview she demonstrated a growing age-appropriate curiosity and seductiveness, indicating that there was "more" she could tell me. There may be one aspect of rigidity in her personality structure—a kind of pseudomaturity and joviality around issues of some importance to her, such as her relationship with her brother. She may be slightly overinvested in her competition with her mother as well. These are subtleties in her drama, however, which in themselves do not detract from the fundamental structural integrity and flexibility of her personality.

Her concerns consisted of a variety of age-appropriate issues ranging across negative and positive affects and across Oedipal and early latency themes.

FORMULATIONS FOR CASE 5

In Steve's case we observe suggestions of severe compromises in the organic integrity of ego functioning, as evidenced by possible sensory (tactile) overreactivity, the immature gross and fine motor integration, receptive and expressive language difficulties, gait, posturing, intermittent perseveration, and overall concrete style of relating. Further testing, including possibly psychological and neurological examinations, would provide important additional data. It would be important to make certain that these severe compromises were not due primarily to anxiety.

The basic ego functions are also seriously compromised, as we observe impairments in regulation of impulses and activity level. A capacity for human relationships is clearly present but severely constricted, as evidenced by the only fleeting and somewhat impersonal concrete way the patient related to the interviewer. While reality testing was intact in a global sense, one would wonder about the potential for regression in reality testing under stress, as evidenced in the "blank look" and rocking on the floor (which may have been a response to anxiety). The narrow range and depth of affect suggest compromises in the flexibility of the personality. The constricted range and depth of thematic communication are further evidence of severe constriction.

Developmentally, he had progressed only to an isolated, somewhat fragmented capacity for representational differentiation around negotiating certain needs ("I want candy") and evidenced significant compromises at all earlier levels.

The overall organization of themes, while not reflecting highly idiosyncratic forms suggestive of a functional psychotic organization, did reflect a much more immature level (a 2½- to 4-year-old level) than would be expected in a 6½-year-old. This immaturity (e.g., islands of thematic concerns rather than cohesive, rich thematic organizations) may be related to an immature capacity for integration based on the compromises in the organic integrity of ego functioning.

We observe a vulnerable ego structure that operates very inflexibly. Nevertheless, we may still observe hints of this child's concerns. After feeling out of control, he attempts to regain control through perseveration and making contact with the interviewer. Frustrated, he becomes angry and out of control again. Yet there are the ambivalent feelings toward the "policeman," again suggesting a desire for regulation and at the same time anger at the source of such regulation. Frightened at his ambivalent ("bad boy") feelings, he shows a momentary loss of relatedness followed by rocking movements. He recovers, however, makes contact again, asking for candy, but then once again becomes angry and out of control. His ability briefly to relate events at school suggests that these concerns permeate his life.

We observe, therefore, how he struggles to deal with his very vulnerable ego functions. The existence of conflicts suggests the basis of motivation for treatment.

FORMULATIONS FOR CASE 6

Both the organic and functional aspects of David's ego structure were age-appropriate, as evinced by his physical and neurological functioning, the quality of his relatedness, his stable mood, and the level of organization of his affects and themes. The flexibility of his personality also seemed age-appropriate. Although one might expect a little more repression of Oedipal concerns by this age, I was quite impressed with his ability to organize his concerns in representational forms and make warm contact with me. During the interview he demonstrated a variety of emotions. He developed a cohesive, organized theme through play with dolls, modulating the emotions of the different characters he created. When his "story" aroused anxiety, he moved on to other—but related—games and themes. Similarly, he showed flexibility in his affect system, though with some limitations.

His main concerns were with anger and conflict (family drama) and not getting enough, although in his interpersonal contact with me he demonstrated the capacity for pleasure and enjoyment as well. While there were concerns with developmentally early (pre-Oedipal) affects, I would guess that these are in an age-appropriate (Oedipal) context. He showed a capacity for a wide variety of affects and did not rely on primitive defenses such as denial, avoidance, and projection; instead, he was able to deal directly with the themes and affects concerning him. In addition, he seemed clever and intelligent, and was able to synthesize, organize, and integrate his material very well. He regulated his behavior in accord with the limits of the playroom (i.e., there was no difficulty with impulse control). He dealt with themes of anger in a displaced way through games. His capacity for pleasure and enjoyment suggested some positive self-esteem. His talk about not getting enough Coke did not seem to be accompanied by a sense of emptiness; rather, it seemed more related to wishes. While there was overall age-appropriate flexibility, there are questions of minor limitations, as indicated both by the absence of more direct themes of pleasure and curiosity and by the subjective feelings of the interviewer regarding limitations in the degree of emotional warmth.

Developmentally, he was fully at the level of representational differentiation with clear mastery of the earlier levels.

His special concerns were reflected in his dramatic rendering of an elaborate family drama, which took up a major part of the session. He was concerned with "things falling off," competition, and being replenished. He may be quite enmeshed in these concerns, trying with some difficulty to gain distance from them in order to resolve them. The question of ego flexibility would seem to depend on how well he works through an intense Oedipal involvement, but there do not seem to be any prominent or major ego restrictions to hamper his resolution. What happens in his family at this time may play a critical role in this resolution. How his family deals with him will in part determine whether he continues developing in an optimal, age-appropriate way.

FORMULATIONS FOR CASE 7

With respect to Joey's basic ego functions, neurological integrity was at the age-appropriate level, as indicated by the quality and level of his motor activity. He seemed relaxed and calm, and his fine and gross motor coordination as well as his language and perceptual-motor ability and coordination all seemed intact. There was a slight lisp to his speech, which was nevertheless understandable.

While reality testing seemed age-appropriate, as did impulse control and affect regulation, there appeared to be a lack of full object constancy in that we did not see if he could function without mother. It was as though he were one step behind the age-appropriate developmental level in his human relationship capacities; flirting, so to speak, with the issues of power and size (phallic issues), but too involved with his dyadic tie to mother to do more than that. His unresolved individuation from mother seemed to be intensified by age-appropriate Oedipal feelings alongside dependent, aggressive, angry, and manipulative themes. He seemed infantile and babyish even with the playful expressions he enjoyed vis-à-vis manipulating mother, who seemed to play right into his hands. I would therefore raise questions about the age-appropriate integrity of the basic ego structure in the line of development related to relationships.

His ego seemed quite rigid, as indicated by his need to maintain the attachment to mother in the playroom, his inability to explore the playroom, his limited ability to relate to me during the course of the interview, and the lack of development of rich themes or organized play. On the positive side, he did elaborate a number of themes and was able to dramatize some of his conflicts around aggression, his tie to mother, his feeling little, and his experience of danger. I felt all this elaboration was in a rather limited context, however.

Predominant affects demonstrated in the interview were apprehension, separation anxiety, and anger, with a facade of playful and pleasurable manipulativeness around the issue of control. The affects thus seemed predominantly representative of earlier age levels (i.e., not at a full Oedipal level). The newness of the situation should not be overlooked, however; he may be capable of other, more flexible affects in a situation familiar to him. Because there seemed to be a hint of warmth and interest in me, as well as some flexibility in the affects as the interview proceeded, there may be some hidden potential in the area of affects; in general, however, the affects seemed rather fixed, rigid, and limited to the pre-Oedipal level.

Joey's anxiety seemed to center on separation, with some

concerns around being engulfed (e.g., the little dog being eaten up), and perhaps some castration anxiety (as evinced by the shooting). Internal signal anxieties did not appear to be fully operable yet in this child's development.

He used avoidance, attempting to avoid me and the playroom situation by a kind of regressive dependent clinging to his mother (it appears from the history that he has been able to go to nursery school and to separate from her at other times). He also made use of projection, as indicated by the degree of fear and apprehension he experienced with regard to the playroom.

He seemed quite apprehensive and frightened of me; he was not prepared to use me in any way as a triangular figure in his life. Although it is possible that he is in a "hot" Oedipal situation, and therefore feels quite frightened of me insofar as I represent the father, I felt that his apprehension stemmed from a lack of *secure* object constancy (i.e., a secure sense of self and a sure grasp of the division between self and others). That he has accomplished this division to some degree was suggested by his general capacity for age-appropriate reality testing and by his ability to regulate affects and impulses. He has not mastered it to the extent expected in a 5-year-old, however; object constancy is a vulnerable area that causes him to regress under stress. His concerns fell somewhere between the pre-Oedipal and Oedipal levels.

He has not fully established himself in an Oedipal configuration—it appeared to frighten him. It was as though he were saying, "I am interested in size, power, and competition, and I want to use my gun" (all early phallic concerns, which lie at the early end of his current developmental phase). At the same time, he did not yet feel secure in his delineation of self. Therefore, he used manipulative devices to maintain a playful, seductive, but dependent tie to mother. From a structural point of view, such devices indicate his lack of readiness for real age-appropriate concerns. Joey therefore employs a stage and a drama that are both one level below his expected developmental level. He has only partially reached an early phase of representational differentiation, often functioning in a representationally fragmented and constricted manner.

FORMULATIONS FOR CASE 8

Basic personality functions were intact, but Warren didn't have age-appropriate ego flexibility. His "stage" was intact; he didn't have any major cracks in it, in terms of reality testing, impulse control, a labile mood, or poor concentration. However, the drama on the stage was not as wide ranging or as full as one would expect at his age. He avoided anger, competition, and sadness. When frustrations built up and he became angry, sad, or embarrassed, he just "chucks it." He used massive avoidance and denial, rather than age-appropriate coping capacities. He used this avoidance whether the disappointment was with friends on the block (e.g., the child who "lies a lot"), his sister being too bossy, or the "work overload" at school. He felt controlled and bossed by two dominating women (mother and older sister) and felt Dad was away too much to be a useful ally.

Compounding his use of avoidance was the fact that Warren is bright, but his short-term memory capacity (auditory-verbal and visual-spatial) is not as good as his reasoning skills. The first six grades will be harder for him than graduate school. For children who are slower on the mechanical, rote memory side, the early grades are the most difficult. Life gets easier for them as creativity, problem-solving, and abstracting abilities become more important. His learning pattern, therefore, further intensified his frustration and anger, leading to massive avoidance. He used avoidance rather globally (e.g., school, friends, and family issues) and in this way demonstrated a marked degree of ego constriction. Yet, his warmth and available sadness provided openings for further growth.

FORMULATIONS FOR CASE 9

Danny's ego functions were intact in terms of reality testing, partially stable mood, relationship capacity, impulse control, and the ability, when not anxious, to focus and concentrate. Under pressure or stress his thinking came overloaded and fragmented. He was able, however, to describe this process. His self-observation capacity indicated that the fragmentation is probably only a transient phenomenon associated with intense anxiety. In terms of constrictions in his basic ego structure, he showed a capacity for warmth and for some affects and themes but not others. When it came to themes of competition and anger, he often felt overloaded and paralyzed. He felt devastated by themes of loss and emptiness. There was also the tendency to feel dominated by his need to be the center of everything and a difficulty in finding a synthesis between the need to be the center of everything and the tendency to feel overwhelmed and alone. There were, therefore, constrictions in the flexibility of age-appropriate ego functions.

We would expect a 10-year-old to be better able to balance the need to be the center and the need also to be part of and have a role in the peer group. We would also expect him to be able to better synthesize and integrate his conflict between being competitive on the one hand and fearful of loss or disappointment on the other. It is difficult to compete without being prepared at times, to lose or experience a disappointment. When one can't experience disappointment, the competition can feel overwhelming and frightening because one can't bear its consequences. Competition for Danny was a life-and-death struggle, rather than one in which there can be momentary and relative winners and losers each day or in each context. For him the competition was not part of a larger relationship pattern. His unusual gift for being alert to even the most subtle emotional nuances in interactions further overwhelmed him, suggesting the possibility of sensory overreactivity.

There were also hints of internal conflicts that were contributing to his character pattern and limitations. As indicated above, he felt conflicted between his need to be the "center" and his fear of loss, as well as his fear of feeling overwhelmed by anger and competition. Within the family, he saw his mother as someone who can't accept his mean and competitive side, even though he perceived these traits in his mother. He perceived father as unavailable, critical, and demanding. He certainly presented as a person who wants to be in the middle of the Oedipal drama, but it was as though he couldn't bear to put too many toes in the water before he got scared and felt overwhelmed, fearful of the competition and loss. In this context, there is a question about his emerging sexual identity in relation to where he is in the Oedipal drama (positive or negative configuration). More data will be needed to explore this issue, however.

It is possible that he had a sense of minimal nurturing support from both parents and that this feeling contributed to his insecurity and, at the same time, to his expectant and grand desires. Both parents were perceived as critical and/or intrusive, rather than giving, only increasing his anxiety over his own expectations.

Another special feature of his ego structure related to the fact that he was aware of so many of his conflicts, fears, and family dynamics. Why, then, was he having so much difficulty? What he could not do was put the pieces together. He saw many trees but not the forest. Many bright, verbal, sensitive adults and children give an impression of great awareness of their inner lives, but this awareness, in some instances, is of only some isolated feelings, not the whole pattern.

Therefore we see in this youngster signs of relatively intact basic ego structure, but also signs of constrictions in ego flexibility, where feelings of fragmentation, global anxiety, and "everyone is my enemy" repeat themselves in many situations. There are also indications of a number of underlying conflicts.

FORMULATIONS FOR CASE 10

This 7-year-old girl with many basic ego functions intact had mastered a number of the early levels of ego development. However, Alice evidenced a deficit in circumscribed areas of representational differentiation (the ability to form categories of experience). Whether this was a regression due to stress or whether she was never fully differentiated was to be determined. From a functional point of view, there was a lack of full differentiation in the area of reality/fantasy. It was, however, circumscribed and not fragmenting to the rest of her personality. There was, therefore, a circumscribed deficit in a basic ego function.

Because of her many assets and intact aspects to her ego functioning, she should do very well in a comprehensive, intensive psychotherapeutic program. (Three or four times a week often works very well in helping a child shore up this kind of deficit.) The therapeutic work must approach from the side of the ego to help her organize her thinking, eventually getting to the types of emotions and affects that are disorganizing. In such a case, one would clearly want to rule out physical contributions, acute or chronic. One would also want to rule out traumatic or abusive experiences. In this case, there were ongoing, severely dysfunctional family patterns.

FORMULATIONS FOR CASE 11

Zachary's basic ego functions, in terms of reality testing, impulse control, concentration, and stable mood, were age-appropriate. There were constrictions in terms of the range and flexibility of his age-appropriate functions. A subtle aspect of these constrictions was the degree to which themes were elaborated without attempts to integrate, connect, or differentiate them. While evidencing reality-testing abilities, he was involved in a great deal of polarized thinking (e.g., idealizations and fragmented ideation). There were also considerable conflicts. He was concerned with aggression, anxiety about his body being hurt, his penis hurting or being hurt, and the need to protect it or patch it up. He also felt very close to his mother, who is beautiful, and he wanted to be beautiful like her. He was also, however, worried about angry witches.

To what degree is his character pattern an expression of conflict over aggression, competition, and castration anxiety related to his relationship with his father? How much do his character patterns relate to expressing ambivalent longings for an idealized mother—to be like mother and close to mother is to be beautiful like her and to deny the scary, evil witches (mother can look depressed, angry, and unavailable at times). I suspect both of these issues are involved. He evidenced conflicts at a number of developmental levels (his father was not very involved with him in his early years, feeling that he was "pushed away by mother"). The developmental history, which cannot be described here, had many elements in it that were likely contributors to his current patterns. It is also appropriate to raise questions about physical or biological contributions to Zachary's emerging character patterns. While considering the factors that may contribute, it is important to keep in mind that this child evidences considerable assets in terms of his intact areas of ego functioning. His ability to engage, interact, and represent experience provides him, with appropriate therapeutic help, the potential to resolve many of his conflicts and form a more flexible and integrated ego structure.

FORMULATIONS FOR CASE 12

From the interview data alone it appeared that there were compromises in the organic integrity of Mark's ego, as seen in his motor patterns and capacity to focus and attend. Mark's basic ego functions were clearly disordered and far below age expectations. The capacities that one would expect to see in a 4½-year-old (i.e., impulse regulation, reality testing, and the capacity to organize affect and thematic communications) were lacking in this child. Rather, as indicated earlier, in terms of these basic ego functions, Mark seemed to be functioning more like a 1- to 2-year-old and, at that, a 1- to 2-year-old who was on a disordered pathway. For example, a healthy 15-month-old child can develop organized nonverbal play themes, something this child could not do. Although one would want further data from psychological testing, one might hypothesize that aspects of Mark's intellectual functioning are actually at the appropriate age level, as evinced by his capacities to spell and name objects. His ability to use his intellect to organize his social and emotional pursuits, however, would appear to be highly compromised by the severe disruption in his basic ego functions, as outlined above.

He seemed to be struggling with the most fundamental issues of early development—namely, the abilities to organize intentional communication, to begin modulating some of his impulses, to begin integrating some aspects of positive and negative feelings, and to begin a better integration of motor functioning and sensorimotor coordination and construct representations. One would expect a child to achieve such developmental tasks by the end of his second year of life. On the basis of this initial playroom interview, therefore, one would recommend a thorough neurological examination. It would not be surprising, however, if such examination revealed only subtle soft signs, as already evinced by his motor patterns and clumsiness; the major findings would be the severe lag in social and emotional development. From this perspective, much of Mark's functioning was below the level of a 2-year-old, whose developmental tasks center on themes of separation, modulation of aggressive impulses, organiza-tion of communication patterns, stabilization of mood, and devel-opment of purposeful initiative.

To round out the evaluation of such a child one would cer-tainly need a detailed developmental history, additional interviews, psychological testing, a neurological exam, and an occupational ther-apy evaluation. The initial clinical interview data alone, however, were enough to indicate serious compromises in all aspects of basic ego functioning.

FORMULATIONS FOR CASE 13

First Interview

My impression was that the physical and neurological com-ponents of Molly's ego functioning were basically intact. There were no obvious signs of disorganization or fragmentation: she showed a reality orientation to the playroom; she modulated and regulated her impulses; she organized her themes. There was no highly inappro-priate affect, but at the same time, the degree of her inhibition, cou-pled with the severe constriction of her affect, made one wonder if there were some fine cracks in the basic ego functions. Molly's drama was evinced in her affect hunger, constriction, and inhibition around age-appropriate themes.

With respect to the flexibility of her basic personality patterns, we observed an extraordinarily rigid little girl, especially for one 4½ years old. One expects rich, complex, organized affects and themes from a child of that age; instead, we saw severe rigidity. Again, the question that should be raised is, Was this constriction covering some below-age-appropriate basic ego functioning? Were there some fine cracks in the structure?

Because there was some question in my mind after the first interview about whether Molly was functioning with characterological constrictions or whether some basic ego functions were indeed well below the age-appropriate level, a second diagnostic interview is pre-sented. In most cases, more than one diagnostic interview is helpful.

Second Interview

During the second interview Molly showed that the hypothesis of "fine cracks in the basic ego functions" suggested by the first interview was not, in fact, the case. She showed that she possessed a greater capacity and range of affect, thematic involvement, and relatedness than she originally revealed. She did, however, confirm the presence of a fundamental constriction in the flexibility of her personality. She continued to communicate in a restrictive, depressed way; her mood was tense, and she showed a restricted range of effects. She developed her themes of aggression in a deep and rich fashion—showing her preoccupation with aggressiveness—and was not involved in the more pleasurable, curious, and sexual aspects of her development, which would have been appropriate for her age. She was quite representational and differentiated, but with intense concerns, conflicts, and anxiety.

The drama that she was dealing with in the context of her inflexible and constricted ego structure revealed itself more clearly during the second interview. She was, in fact, preoccupied with themes of aggression. She made it clear that she was concerned with hurting and being hurt; that she saw her emerging femininity as caught up in this aggressive theme and therefore too laden with conflict to handle; and that she was quite uncomfortable with the picture of herself as a "poisonous snake." She associated the snake picture with a fear of being overwhelmed and "not breathing," but took reassurance from a demanding, *concrete* connectedness with the significant others in her life.

Therefore, in summary, we see a picture of a 4½-year-old girl whose ego functioning is already highly constricted and whose conflicts center on very primitive themes of aggression, being overwhelmed, and losing important objects in her life.

FORMULATIONS FOR CASE 14

There are questions about Eddie's gait. While he showed a grasp of the reality of the playroom and was organized and intentional in his gestures and preverbal sense of reality, his capacity to organize thinking at an age-appropriate level did seem compromised, as shown by his fragmented verbal communication. Similarly, although he showed no overt signs of impulse control problems, one would wonder whether he has difficulty controlling his impulses in other settings, given his preoccupation during the interview with twisting off the dolls' arms and otherwise hurting the dolls. Given these observations, plus the poverty of the range and depth of his symbolic communications (themes), one might postulate that Eddie's emerging self-representation is itself compromised in terms of being an organizational unit that provides stability for basic personality functions, such as reality testing, impulse regulation, mood stabilization, and an ever-growing delineation of self from nonself. Again, the fact that we did not see major disruptions in all these personality functions indicates that we were dealing with partial difficulties, most notably at the representational level.

For a 3½-year-old boy, he functioned well below his age level in capacities, such as organizing communication and affect, and expressing a richness and depth of affect. That he was so tense and apprehensive, showed such a narrow range of affect, and only meagerly developed his themes suggest the degree to which his personality structure is significantly "walled off." Thus, we see that he is already using major characterological constrictions to hold together what would appear to be a fragile personality organization. Developmentally, he has progressed in a constricted manner to a level of representational elaboration, but not fully to a level of representational differentiation.

Observations of his thematic sequence and affect gave a picture of some of his developmental concerns. He has been struggling with his ambivalence, and particularly with his angry feelings. He has not given up on the human world; indeed, he is beginning to work out a compromise that features a pattern of impersonal relatedness.

In sum, we see a child who is invested in the world and wants to relate to others. He can use gestures and fragmented verbal phrases to communicate somewhat intentionally. He cannot, however, organize his representational world. Fragments of aggressive imagery dominate. He therefore evidences a deficit in a core of ego function— the capacity to organize and differentiate representational experience. Additional interview and developmental evaluations were indicated to provide a fuller picture of Eddie's uneven development.

FORMULATIONS FOR CASE 15

The physical and neurological aspects of Jane's basic ego functions seemed intact, as indicated by her gross and fine motor activity, language ability, and overall intellectual skills (evinced by her capacity to name the letters and pick the correct letter for her sister's name, copy circles, etc.). She also showed an overall awareness of what was going on and exhibited a capacity to follow instructions and to focus her attention in an extraordinarily effective manner in the course of the play.

With regard to the psychological aspects of basic ego functions, Jane seemed at an age-appropriate level in her ability to organize her thematic communication. She presented her descriptions and occasional interactive themes in a cohesive, organized way. Her affect, while chronically anxious and apprehensive, was nonetheless well organized and integrated with her thematic presentation. She also displayed a fundamental capacity for a relatedness infused with personal warmth; her relatedness was in the age-appropriate range. Her self-modulated activity level, impulse control, and understanding of the situation were all consistent with age-appropriate capacities. As indicated, her mood was stable, albeit constricted in range. Jane's basic ego functions, therefore, seemed to be at an age-appropriate level.

In terms of her flexibility, however, she showed a number of marked constrictions not appropriate for her age, particularly with regard to the range of affect. We would expect that Jane—being close to 3 years old—would demonstrate gleeful pleasure, assertiveness, curiosity, and, in the appropriate situation, signs of aggression or negativism, all in the symbolic and representational mode. Jane showed little of this affective range. Although some mild aggressiveness was seen in the interactive play with the fish, the affect accompanying it was weak and pale. Of even greater concern, there were few signs of joyful pleasure, and while there was some capacity for exploring and moving around the room, here, too, there seemed to be some constriction. In addition, the affects were not developed in a deep, rich manner consistent with age expectations.

Similarly, her thematic development lacked range and her themes lacked richness and depth. As a child moves from age 2 to age 3, one should see a greater capacity than Jane showed to use the representational mode to convey inner feelings, thoughts, and wishes; this development parallels a readiness to depart from the strictly descriptive level wherein the child names objects. This developmental progression was not evident in Jane's communications with her mother, which were permeated with apprehension and a generally tense quality. Jane's preference for the descriptive level was more consistent with the style of a 2- to 2½-year-old than with that of an almost 3-year-old. In sum, the flexibility of the personality was markedly below age-appropriate capacity, resembling that of a tense and anxious 2- to 2½-year-old.

With respect to this child's concerns, we can only speculate about what might be responsible for the constriction in thematic and affective range and depth. We saw that both she and mother seemed to be chronically apprehensive and tense, and that when Jane experimented with aggression, taking the fish to bite mother, mother quickly turned the tables. Although mother smiled (superficially and tensely) and tried to make this turnabout part of the game, her "quick trigger" suggested to me that she was not comfortable with Jane's emerging capacity for organized assertiveness and exploration and their aggressive components. Additional supportive evidence for this possibility was Jane's tendency to stay physically close to mother and hold onto her, as opposed to being more comfortable with the explorativeness that would accompany her otherwise confident cognitive development. Though a fundamental warmth was evident in their relatedness, so was an underlying uneasiness. Regarding separation, explorativeness, and aggression, it would seem that at one time in their relationship there was a greater capacity for shared pleasure, which is now on more tenuous grounds, caught up in anxiety.

In summary, then, we see a child of 2 years and 11 months whose basic ego functions are intact, but who seems to have severe constrictions in age-appropriate flexibility of personality functions and perhaps is conflicted and concerned with the issues of separation, assertion, and aggression. Using our metaphor, Jane's stage is structurally intact in its physical, neurological, and psychological ego functions, but it is already developing some major constrictions. These constrictions are probably responsible for some of the symptoms that caused this child to be brought in for the evaluation.

The interview was conducted with the mother in the playroom because the child was so young. I did not try to have Jane come in alone, although she might have been able to, particularly after spending some time with me and her mother in the waiting room. With children this young, one learns a great deal about the child by watching his or her interactions with mother, although one may wish to know how a child like Jane would communicate with the clinician without mother present in a follow-up interview (if the child was comfortable separating from mother). Jane's interview thus differs from the interviews of the older children presented here, where most of the children were in the playroom with me alone.

FORMULATIONS FOR CASE 16

The clinical impression of Sam was of a child who at age 3 years was significantly delayed in organizing a number of basic ego functions. He was not yet at a representational level and only evidenced early forms of intentional gestural communication (sometimes variably). At the same time, he seemed emotionally comfortable with closeness and dependency, but didn't have flexibility to negotiate a new relationship comfortably or deal with a full range of 10- to 16-month-old level affects and behaviors. His ability to concentrate and modulate behavior was variable.

Contributing to his deficit in basic ego functioning was a marked receptive and expressive language delay, fine (e.g., fisted a crayon and scribbled diffusely) and gross motor delays, and indications of sensory reactivity and sensory processing difficulties. He was between 1 and 2 years behind in terms of his functional capacities. Normally, we would see representational capacities emerging between 18 and 24 months. He had some splinter skills and scatter in certain areas.

After further observation of Sam confirmed these preliminary impressions, it became clear that he required additional evaluations including

1. Language evaluation by a speech pathologist (including hearing by an audiologist), with the possibility of two or more sessions a week of language work.
2. A sensory and motor evaluation by an occupational therapist, to look for sensory reactivity and sensory processing difficulties, with the possibility of one to two sessions a week of work.
3. A neurologic and pediatric evaluation to assess possible organic contributions.
4. A parent and family evaluation with the possibility of following through with counseling for the parents to help them set up a home program and deal with their own emotional reactions and patterns.
5. An evaluation for interactive play therapy, with the possibility of three to five sessions a week.
6. Consideration of a psychoeducational preschool program.

A marked ego deficit in a very young child, while obviously challenging, is also an opportunity to pinpoint the specific nature of the child's uneven development and plan a comprehensive and intensive program of clinical work.

FORMULATIONS FOR CASE 17

Leah's basic personality and ego functions were at an age-appropriate level in terms of her ability to relate and engage, use gestures intentionally, and use early representational modes consistent with her age. She was able to control impulses, concentrate, and maintain a relatively even mood, at least in unchallenging situations. At the same time, there were indications of a rather marked constriction in the range of affect she had available: She evidenced no pleasure, and showed no spontaneity and very little creativity. Her gross motor coordination was age-appropriate, but she was about 2 months behind on fine motor coordination.

It appeared, therefore, that she showed constrictions in the flexibility of her age-appropriate personality functions with a narrowing of the range, particularly in the areas of pleasure, joy, and spontaneity. She also would be expected to have difficulties in handling the anger and feelings of emptiness that appeared to be a part of her interaction pattern with her parents. Her parents were compromised in their ability to support a fuller range of affects, behaviors, and emerging representations. The interactions with her parents not only give a picture of their prior relationship, but also of her present and likely continuing interaction patterns. As the representational system forms, experience is becoming symbolized. We have character formation in the making. Leah's emerging personality is defined, in part, by these ongoing interactional patterns. There is, therefore, a unique opportunity to help Leah and her parents negotiate more adaptive representational patterns.

FORMULATIONS FOR CASE 18

Elizabeth evidenced a lag in negotiating the first critical developmental process of shared attention and engagement, in part due to her own constitutional and maturational pattern as well as mother's personality structure. This first developmental process is the beginning of attention and concentration and forming and enjoying relationships, both critical ego functions. Identifying this challenge early led to assisting Elizabeth and her mother and father. They learned to adjust their pattern to Elizabeth's unique maturational pattern and the early stages of ego development were successfully negotiated.

CONCLUDING REMARKS

In concluding this section on formulation, brief mention should again be made of the fact that, in routine clinical care settings, the clinical interview is but one of many sources of data one uses in arriving at a formulation. The foregoing discussion demonstrates the degree to which the clinical interview can be the cornerstone of the formulation. Notwithstanding that observational data derived from the interview setting can be used for arriving at good clinical hypotheses, additional data are always necessary. For example, psychological testing provides valuable information that will enhance one's capacity to make clinical judgments and develop appropriate formulations. It is interesting to note that the observational categories described earlier may also be used to organize the data that emerge from psychological test reports. For example, the findings of the Bender Visual Motor Gestalt Test and various intelligence tests provide very useful data about the physical and neurological integrity of the central nervous system. Subtle lags in instrumental or conceptual cognitive abilities can be picked up through these tests. Data from the Rorschach will occasionally expose a child's covert difficulties in distinguishing fantasy from reality (assuming this distinction is age-appropriate). Responses to the Rorschach, as well as to the TAT and various figure-drawing exercises, also provide exceedingly valuable data on the level of personality development and the types of concerns and/or conflicts a child is experiencing. Indeed, psychological testing can provide important findings regarding all three of the questions we have examined in this chapter: 1) the basic integrity of the personality structure, as evinced by the level of basic organic and psychological ego functions; 2) the flexibility of the personality; and 3) the child's specific concerns and conflicts.

One may also organize psychological test data in terms of the child's developmental level of ego functioning, including the quality of attention and engagement, intentionality and organization, capacity to represent or symbolize affects or emotional themes (and which ones), and ability to categorize and differentiate these in terms of self/non-self, fantasy versus reality, different thematic areas (e.g., dependency versus aggression), and so forth (Greenspan 1989).

One point should be stressed, however. When conducting a full evaluation, a clinician should optimally have specific questions in mind to ask via the psychological testing. In other words, if done systematically and logically, the clinical interview will provide first-order information that raises hypotheses with varying degrees of certainty. (Some questions arise that are more in the nature of hunches than hypotheses.) For example, from the clinical interview one may have questions about whether there is a lag in perceptual-motor integration because the child showed some delay in fine motor coordination and some lack of clarity in speech. Thus a specific question will be formulated for clarification by the diagnostic psychological testing.

Similarly, we may see a child who seems to have good organization of affect and age-appropriate thematic organization but who, once or twice during the interview, seems to bring in a theme from out of left field, or who demonstrates some affects that are far below age expectations or otherwise inappropriate, or who hints at depressive and suicidal themes. In such cases, psychological testing might provide valuable insights about how experience is organized.

Another example is the child who comes across in the interview as unduly polarized, with extreme personality rigidities, and who shows only the passive domain of human experience. Psychological testing may reveal whether a hidden vulnerability or weakness in the fabric of the personality structure underlies this seeming characterological constriction, or whether in different circumstances the child shows greater variation and flexibility in the range of experience.

While traditional psychological testing (including intelligence tests, Rorschachs, TATs, and Bender Visual Motor Gestalt Tests) involves many unstructured exercises (e.g., the Rorschach), it complements the unstructured clinical interview in an important way. Even the most unstructured components of the routine battery employ standard stimuli, and the responses of many children to these stimuli have been studied. Therefore, in addition to enabling us to study certain areas of personality functioning (such as intellectual functioning) in greater depth than is possible in the clinical interview, testing also offers an opportunity to see how a child deals with these standard stimuli.

The above remarks are intended only as passing comments on psychological testing; the present context does not allow a full discussion of all the complex issues that could be raised. The point I want to emphasize, however, is that in a systematic clinical evaluation, the clinical interview should be used as the basis or framework for raising questions. Optimally, clinicians ask highly specific questions via psychological testing, even though they must also be prepared to hear answers to questions that they did not raise.

There are other sources of data that complement the data that emerge from the clinical interview, most important, obviously, are medical and neurological evaluations when indicated. Where there are questions about conceptual or instrumental aspects of intellectual functioning, specialized testing may be appropriate; such testing may range from hearing tests to tests for specific perceptual-motor difficulties, to tests for particular processing difficulties in the verbal or visual-spatial areas. Furthermore, information from the child's regular and special school teachers, as well as information from others who are an important part of the child's life (e.g., at religious school, special clubs, and other activities), are all valuable sources of data, particularly when the clinical interview raises difficult questions.

Therefore, in addition to standard psychological studies, it is important to be aware of specialized studies to pursue specific areas of auditory-verbal processing, visual-spatial processing, fine and gross motor and perceptual motor functioning, sensory reactivity and processing, and selected aspects of cognitive and language functioning. Occupational therapy and speech pathology, as well as medical and neurological evaluations, must also be considered.

In this work, we will not be able to consider these other sources of information. We will, however, briefly consider information that one should routinely obtain from parents about parental and family functioning as well as the child's developmental history.

7

Interviewing the Parents: Selected Comments

IN THIS CHAPTER I will discuss aspects of the clinical interview with the parents, including observing each parent's personality organization, noting family patterns, obtaining a developmental history, conveying your recommendations, and helping parents deal with resistances and/or other factors that may interfere with their "hearing" or following through on your recommendations. These subjects will not be discussed comprehensively. Rather, some suggestions on selected aspects of interviewing the parents will be covered.

ASSESSING THE PARENTS

The same basic method that we used to assess the child will be used to assess the parents, namely, systematic observations made during an unstructured interview. These firsthand observations constitute the most reliable information you can get about the parents, so you must make the most of the interview period by way of facilitating communication. It is especially important during the opening moments not to lead the parents. During this initial phase, focus first on the parents as individuals, observing each person as a clinical entity, and focus second on their relationship.

Using the same principles used in the interview with the child, I try to let the parents start the interview while I listen. At the beginning of the typical interview, I will be warm and clearly available; I make eye contact, smile, nod or shake hands when appropriate, and then look expectant. I assume that the parents know why they are here and I will not patronize them, even inadvertently, by structuring the beginning. In these circumstances most people wish to, and will, structure things for themselves. They will say, for example, that the reason they have come is that Johnny is having problems in school, or Sally is having nightmares and disturbing the whole family, or some such broad statement. If they look anxious for some moments as they greet me and sit down, I will patiently allow them time to organize their thoughts rather than doing it for them. I will not say, e.g., "Well, obviously you've come to tell me about Johnny. You've already told me on the phone. . . . " Rather, I want to see what the parents do with the situation.

Depending on the situation, I might say, for example, "You are looking at me very expectantly," to which they could respond, "We were thinking you might have a lot of questions." Then I might say, "I probably will, but I don't know where to begin. I'd like to hear from you first." Given permission in this way, they will be off and running. If they seem especially anxious in the first few minutes I might say, "Sometimes it's hard to get one's thoughts together in a situation like this," which may serve to relax them and help them organize their thinking without deflecting attention from the purpose of the interview.

The parents usually begin with something related to the child. But they may begin with family issues, their discomfort about coming to see you, or more tangential issues. They may start with one sentence about the child and then switch to their own parents or some problems at work; 10 minutes later you still have not heard anything more about the child. Rather than interrupting or bringing them back to their starting point, it is preferable in such circumstances to follow the parents' natural associative trends.

For example, the father may be talking about some argument he had with his boss. Listen carefully to this aggressive theme and ask yourself if it is related to how the parents feel about coming to see you. You may hypothesize that they are expecting some competition or rivalry. If the parental theme focuses on being humiliated, the parents may be fearful of exposing something. Alternatively, if they have never talked to a psychiatrist before, they may have some unusual ideas about what is going to happen, such as a fantasy that they are going to tell you about their child and you are going to take the child away and lock them up. If you feel some strong affect at the beginning, or if the opening moves are not in the range that you usually encounter, it is worthwhile to ask an open-ended question that plays back in a supportive way—not in an intrusive or guilt-provoking way—what you have noticed.

The amount of work you have to do at the beginning of the interview says something about the family structure. Highly tangential material offered at the beginning of the interview may reflect resistance and fearfulness. Often your supportive feedback can help some anxiety to emerge and thus make it easier for parents to tell their story. Let me emphasize, however, that you make such comments only after you have had an opportunity to observe the parents for a few minutes and have listened to the content and sequence of their associative trends. In this way you will get a clear picture of the issues the parents are trying to deal with and thus be able to form questions or comments which more precisely reflect their concerns.

For example, a couple came to see me about a young adolescent boy. They looked at each other, they looked at me, and I looked back. We went through an uncomfortable few moments that allowed quick access to the fact that they did not easily give me anything, as they did not give much to their teenage son. Eventually it emerged that the parents were very depressed; they were caught up in marital problems and rarely talked to each other; the father was also having terrible troubles at work. Having heard about these issues, I was able to ask specific questions that would help them elaborate their concerns.

To assess the parents in this initial phase, I use the same categories that I described earlier for observing children. That is, I observe their physical makeup, neurological integrity, gross and fine motor systems, sensory modalities, speech, activity levels, etc. Then I observe their mood and affects; the way they organize their thinking, communications, and affects. From all these observations I learn something about their personality structures and can make a good guess as to their degree of pathology; that is, whether they are in the neurotic range, the characterological range, or the borderline psychotic range.

I am also thinking developmentally about the sequence of their verbal communications, observing whether they are attentive and engaged, gesturing intentionally, able to elaborate their concerns in a representational form (i.e., using words), able to differentiate their concerns (i.e., present them in a logical manner). I am also observing constrictions. What themes or concerns are missing (e.g., Why are the parents only concerned about discipline and not warmth and closeness?).

In addition to observing each parent individually, it is important to see how they relate to each other and how, as a team, they relate to you. You want to look at who dominates, and how they share in telling their concerns. Watching the evolution of their story can give you some answers. For instance, some parents can give you a rich, organized history of the family and impression of the child's problem. These people show you that they operate together in a fairly organized, cohesive manner. Other parents, in contrast, may keep undermining one another, causing the history of the child's difficulties to evolve in a fragmented, disorganized way. Tangential thinking gives you a picture of a disorganized family environment.

It is also important to observe their perceptions of one another. For example, take a case where the wife saw the husband as a big tyrant (he was, in fact, 6'4") and herself as a helpless, dependent little thing who could run the family only by stealthy manipulation because she could not deal directly with his explosiveness. The couple had stereotyped images of each other which were based on their experiences with their own families. After further discussion, it turned out that the father actually felt very dependent and insecure and was frightened that his wife would leave him. In fact, after a series of interviews it emerged that the mother realized she had the power in the family. She became aware that she identified to some degree with her own father, who was a very strong figure in her family, and that she had taken on certain of his controlling characteristics. As this couple saw that their perceptions of each other were partly based on projections of certain stereotyped images, they became more flexible in the way they related to each other. It was useful to understand these projections because both were also projecting a denied part of their selves onto their son, who had psychosomatic difficulties.

Third, it is important to look at the specific way each parent relates to, and what each feels about, the child. Often you can pick this up by letting each parent describe the child's problem without your asking many questions. Listen to their associative trends. In particular, you want to look for distorted perceptions, which play an important role in the child's pathology.

For example, with a number of boys there is a father who sees the child as a threat (a revival of Oedipal issues). Afraid of his own aggression, the father remains somewhat distant and aloof. Mother, on the other hand, sees the child as a passive, dependent thing whom she needs to nurture. The parents paint two very different pictures: one talks about the child as helpless and dependent, and the other talks about the child as an aggressive monster. Although quite discordant, these may be firmly fixed perceptions.

Of particular interest is to what degree these distorted perceptions of the child reflect displacements from problems that the parents are having with each other. Frequently the child becomes the receptacle for problems that the parents cannot work out. Mother may have some impulses that she would like to relate to father but cannot, and instead deflects them onto the child. Father may feel quite angry at and threatened by mother, and may deflect these feelings onto the child.

In one family, for example, mother was somewhat insecure in her ability to take an assertive, affectionate role with her husband, seeing him as aloof, withdrawn, and absorbed in his legal practice. She was always complaining that he did not pay attention to her. Meanwhile, when it came time to make love, she was always a little withdrawn and would find excuses. Mother defended against some of her warm feelings toward her husband by seeing him as cold, aloof, and uninterested, and then transferred some of the warmth from her own instinctual interests onto her 5-year-old boy. Her discomfort with the Oedipal aspects of this situation, however, involved her in a defensive strategy. She avoided some of her warm feelings with "heated," intense power struggles with this child. Here, one can see that mother perceived her husband as cold (he was actually much warmer than she thought) in order to protect herself against her feelings. She used the child as the object of some of her feelings. The child's response to the struggle was to hold onto his feces (having bowel movements about once every 10 days) and show negativism. He was basically locked, both characterologically and instinctually, into an early pattern, even though there were some signs that he had reached an Oedipal phase of development.

In such a situation, it is important to see that a child is more than a victim; he or she may have played an important role in initiating the family pattern. By the time children are 5 or 6, they have their own needs and intentions and may take advantage of a particular family situation to promote these. In some families where the parents are having difficulties, one child will get right in the middle and want to solve all their problems, while another will say, "The heck with it, let them struggle" and tune out the family in favor of greater involvement with school and friends. To be sure, even the latter child suffers some effects of the parental dynamics, but they may have less impact and stay with him for a shorter period of time because he does not essentially "buy into" them. In other words, he does not see parental difficulties as an opportunity to satisfy some of his instinctual needs. He thinks the parental battles are confusing, and more or less tunes them out, seeking to meet certain needs elsewhere.

In looking at the parents' conscious and unconscious perceptions of the child, it is important to learn how these views relate to the child's developmental stage. Although some parents have fixed, distorted perceptions of the child, these may nevertheless be less undermining at certain stages than others. The father who sees his young latency-aged son as a narcissistic extension of his own athletic abilities may spend a lot of time with his child, who, if lucky, may love sports and enjoy learning new skills. Dad's overcontrol is therefore tolerable. But this same attitude may impede the child's strivings at other phases of development, such as adolescence.

The engulfing mother who sees all children as helpless and dependent may be an excellent parent in the first months of her child's life, since infants basically need a special kind of love and care. However, when the child gets to be 12 to 16 months old and starts walking around the house, wanting to explore and separate, you may see such a mother continually undermining both the child's exploratory activities and his sense of mastery or real separation from her. The mother's undermining may take one of numerous forms, such as anger, control, or manipulation, all of which may serve to keep the child at an infantile level.

In families where the mother and father are not living together, each one can still offer support in the treatment process. There may also be other family members or surrogate family members who are crucial to the child. Have them come in and contribute to the initial diagnostic process by sharing their impression of the child; they can be helpful not only as informants but also as supports of the child during treatment. For instance, you may want to involve a neighborhood friend who is the major babysitter for the 5-year-old while mother works. Although you need to work clinically through the mother, this surrogate mother definitely needs to be taken into account.

In summary, during the first part of the interview, focus your attention on structural personality issues and family dynamics. Do not be too concerned with whether the parents get right to the point of why they called. If they start off on a tangent, let that go on for a while because it will give you a good picture of what kind of people they are and how they relate to each other. Be on the lookout for parental perceptions and possible distortions in the context of the child's age-appropriate developmental activities. One or both parents may have a character disorder or some neurotic configurations that distort the way the child is perceived. Then, after the first 20 minutes or so, you may want to move in and structure the interview in order to get a more detailed picture of what is going on in the family and of the current problems and overall development of the child in question.

THE PRESENTING PROBLEM

Follow up whatever statements the parents have made about why they came to see you with questions that elicit a clear picture of the child's current problems. Ask for examples of each and every problem and inquire about its manifestation in all the child's environments: at school, at home, on the block with friends, and so on.

Find out exactly when each problem began and what precipitated it, e.g., a family crisis, a certain event, the child's (or his family's) conflicts about his development.

Your goal is to obtain a brief history and complete cross-sectional picture of the "present illness" and overall functioning. Thus, you require details about the child's current functioning and his functioning just before the precipitating events *in each area outlined in the categories of Chapter 2.* A detailed knowledge of the child's functioning across the board requires great patience and systematic focusing (i.e., on each category). It will, however, tell you about *all* the problem areas, all the areas of strength and coping, and their contexts. This sort of detailed history is crucial to your fully understanding not only the current problems, their likely precipitants, and their pervasiveness, but also the related strengths and vulnerabilities. Knowing about the child's relationships with adults and peers, mood, affects, anxieties, and interests and concerns is important no matter what the problem is.

Sometime in the first or second interview, it may be helpful to outline the steps in the clinical assessment process and explain the importance of each step, such as hearing about their concerns, doing a developmental history, learning about the family, and talking to and playing with the child. Pay special attention to the parents' ideas about the necessity of each step and explore their thinking as a way to understand the family. Avoid power struggles and keep exploring if there are different ideas about how best to proceed.

Often at the end of the first or second interview, parents will ask what they should tell their child about his or her upcoming session with the clinician. First, listen to the parents' own ideas about how to prepare their child. Help them reason about the child's developmental capacity as a way to decide how and what to discuss with the child. Sometimes it is best to help the child see the process as a way the family can understand its feelings and relationships better. If a child himself or herself recognizes a clear challenge, it may be useful for him or her to anticipate receiving some assistance in meeting the challenge. Since the clinical interview should be a helpful and at times enjoyable experience for the child, helping the parents understand how you will talk and play with the child is always helpful.

TAKING THE HISTORY

In addition to the routine questions one asks in taking a history to elicit information in the biological, physical, and nutritional realms, you must also obtain information about the child's psychological development. Parents vary in their ability to be good historians, particularly with regard to this latter aspect of their child's life. You can help by asking the right kinds of questions.

Your questioning should facilitate an understanding of how the child came to be the way he is, i.e., what constitutional and/or experiential factors were involved. The clinician who knows how normal development progresses should be able to discover whether the child always had certain tendencies, or whether he functioned well and then suddenly began having difficulties or regressed. By obtaining data relevant to each of the observational categories (see Chapter 2) from birth onward, you will have a picture of when the child's problems began and perhaps some clues about what caused them. The developmental table in Chapter 3 is useful in this context; it shows both the range of normal behavior for each age group and the important developmental milestones. Proceed systematically from the time the family began considering having a child, through the pregnancy and delivery, up to the present age of the child. For each period you want to make sure you know something about the neurological and physiological aspects, the psychological development, the interpersonal development, and important events and patterns in the family's life. As you can well imagine, taking a history properly may require more than one session. Begin your history-taking with a sketch of the family tree in terms of the presence or absence of mental illness, learning disorders, and chronic physical illnesses. Then inquire about the mother's prenatal experiences, finding out about nutrition, drugs, emotional stress, and her feelings and her husband's about the pregnancy. Ask too about their experience of the birth process itself.

Although you want to know something about each area of development as outlined in Table 3-1, there are certain basic developmental tasks on which you can focus your questions. To begin with, you should get an impression of the baby's capacity to establish the basic homeostatic patterns early in life. The key issues here are regulation of and interest in the world, which depend in part on the maturity of the baby's central nervous system and/or special sensitivities or hyperreactions to auditory, visual, and tactile stimuli, as well as the baby's own movement patterns. Some babies quiet down as soon as they see the mother or hear her voice. Other babies need to be rocked and touched in just the right way to reach a stage of equilibrium. In the latter case you want to understand the cause of the child's hypersensitivity: for example, was there an immaturity in the child's central nervous system? Or might the child have been colicky, with an allergy to dairy products? Ask about the baby's environment as well. In sum, you want to get a picture of the initial organization of the central nervous system, which is indicated in part by the infant's ability to establish organized patterns, to interrelate these patterns with mother's patterns, to regulate the self, and to become engaged in the world by being alert for reasonable periods of time.

Early individual differences can now be clinically assessed in the newborn period and during the first year of life. Early regulatory differences may contribute to later patterns (Brazelton 1973; DeGangi and Greenspan 1988b, 1989; Greenspan 1989).

Continuing with the newborn phase, you also want to get a feeling for the mother's response to the infant and vice versa. First, was an attachment or relationship formed between the two, and what was its quality? You want to see the richness and depth of that capacity to form relationships, the kind of emotions, and whether the mother's feelings were predominantly negative or positive.

If an attachment was formed and you know something about its quality, next find out about the quality of the infant's beginning capacity to become intentional and initiate interactions, such as pointing or reaching out to be picked up, and how well the parents "read"and responded to these signals in all the emotional domains (e.g., dependency, assertiveness). You want to look at this capacity for interaction in terms of both the motoric elements of the sensorimotor system and the human elements—that is, the baby's capacity to see the caregiver as a person with whom to interact and from whom to get feedback. You want to get a picture of what the process was like for this particular child. Was this a mother who, every time the child pushed back to get a better look, held the child in because she felt rejected? Or was this a mother who, as soon as the child showed any curiosity, threw the child off her lap and said, "There, go it alone"?

The capacity for balanced empathy on the part of the nurturing figure—that is, the ability to be indulgent, giving, loving, and protective, and at the same time to experience emotionally something of what the infant experiences—is essential. A mother with balanced empathy is both in tune with her infant and able to distinguish her own needs from her infant's needs. A father who consistently projects onto the infant and smothers him with care may be able to support development for the first couple of months, but may make it hard for the infant when he begins to become more intentional in the middle of his first year.

Toward the end of the first year of life, one of the infant's major developmental tasks, which is a part of his general growing ability for intentional two-way communication, is to learn to distinguish between and differentiate the different people in the environment; particularly, to learn the difference between the people who have been giving him primary care versus other people. Stranger anxiety is only *one* of many possible signs of that capacity. Some infants show almost no stranger anxiety and yet have highly integrated differentiating capacities, which early in life include an unusually high degree of trust. These babies might have a big smile for mother rather than fear or anxiety for the stranger. On the other hand, extreme stranger anxiety may represent tension in the infant. Most important is to determine whether enough differentiation occurred for the infant to engage in reciprocal communication patterns (i.e., purposeful, causal interactions) in a range of emotional domains. In your history-taking with the parents, you want to get a picture of how the child fared at learning these early tasks.

You want to find out whether, as the child began his second year of life, he developed more organized behavioral and emotional patterns. The advances at this time are part of the more general capacity for organizing behaviors and affects and using gestures to communicate intentionally. They include stringing together many cause-and-effect units of behavior into a complex pattern. These complex patterns serve emotional goals such as running to the door when Daddy comes home, reaching up, giving him a hug, and then putting on his hat and giggling. As part of the toddler's growing behavioral organization, we also see more imitative behavior, greater initiative (e.g., when hungry, the baby may lead mother into the kitchen and point to the refrigerator), responses to limits (e.g., beginning to respond to "No"), the use of distal modes of communication (e.g., affect, vocal, and motor gestures across space are used to communicate such basic messages as satisfaction, annoyance, or pride), and the ability to begin integrating affective priorities. In addition, explore how the child negotiated the beginning of the separation process, practicing the subphase of separaton-individuation (Mahler et al. 1975), and whether he was capable of new and original behavior (tertiary circular reactions) (Piaget 1969).

Next, you want to find out when, and if, the child began displaying the capacity to represent things or experiences mentally. This capacity involves the child's ability to represent or symbolize emotional themes. This representational elaboration should encompass all the emotional domains (dependency, separation, assertiveness, exploraton, curiosity, anger, pleasure, etc.) and is evidenced by both interactive pretend play and language (as used for intentional communication, not just description). Along with this new capacity, one may, because of the greater awareness of the world, see a variety of emotional patterns—joy, excitement, anger, and stubbornness, neediness, etc.

During this stage, the development of object permanence evolves further (Piaget 1969). The child can find an object that has been hidden for more than only a moment. There is a greater capacity for recall and a greater capacity to hold onto experiences over time (i.e., emotional memory).

The emergence of this new symbolic capacity essentially transforms the child. Whereas previously the child was a "behaving being," with only vaguely organized internal experiences, now the child is a thinking being.

During the second and third years, the child continues to elaborate and refine the mental representations of the self and the world. One should ask if the child has further elaborated the representational capacity (i.e., thematic trends at a symbolic level—using words, play objects such as dolls, etc.) in all of life's emotional domains: love, dependency, pleasure, assertion, protest, anger, negativism, etc. If not, note which thematic trends were absent (e.g., no intimacy or no curiosity), and you will see the emergence of character limitations (rigidities).

It is also necessary for the child to differentiate his mental representations. This differentiation may include the child's ability in pretend play to connect elements of the play logically (the rocket is flying because of its powerful motor), or to tie together ideas in conversation. It also involves the child's ability to differentiate or categorize different types of internal experiences, including distinguishing self from nonself and knowing the difference between basic emotional tendencies such as dependency and aggression or constructive assertiveness and destructive anger. This differentiation forms the basis of reality testing and other basic ego functions, such as impulse control, a stable mood, and the ability to concentrate. It is a long process, starting around 20 to 24 months and continuing until age 4 or 5. But by age 3½ to 4, reality testing certainly should be reasonably well established. For instance, at this age, children should be involved in fantasy, but, when you insist, should be able to test reality reasonably well. When you see a 3-year-old who is not moving in this direction, who is unable to differentiate self from nonself at an internal symbolic or representational level, you know that child is having problems.

Referring to children aged 3½ to 4, Mahler and colleagues (1975) describe the attainment of "libidinal object constancy," that is, the capacity of the child to maintain a *constant* delineated representation of self and a *constant* delineated representation of significant loved ones in terms of a mental form or psychological structure. The child who has achieved the stage of libidinal object constancy has a sense of security that she never had before. The child does not need the continuous presence of the parent to feel secure because she can now maintain an inner representation of the parent. This capacity forms the basis of the sense of security. Your questions to the parents should focus on how the child dealt with separations, what happened when she was angry, and what happened when she started going to nursery school. When 3½- and 4-year-olds show an excessive reaction of extreme panic, separation anxieties, or fears of the parents dying or never returning, it may suggest that their capacity for libidinal object constancy is vulnerable.

Up to this point the child has been mainly involved in what can be called dyadic relationship patterns, that is, he sees the environment predominantly as a two-person system composed of himself and a significant other. The significant other is interchangeable, even though the child can distinguish between mother, father, playmates, and others. The key other may switch, but if the key other leaves or is destroyed, then the child has no one else, which is why the child in the dyadic phase experiences feelings like anger, jealousy, and envy as so frightening. With representational differentiation and a stable sense of self, the youngster becomes able to move on—assuming there has been appropriate maturation of the central nervous system—to more complicated triangular relationship patterns, which are characteristic of the phallic-Oedipal phase of development. As the child progresses toward triangular patterns, one also observes shifting interests—in power (rocket ships) and then interests in the body and where babies come from all emerge. These interests alone, however, do not indicate triangular relationships.

What distinguishes the triangular relationship of the Oedipal phase is that the child's relationships have a different style and sophistication. Adding another counter to a game formerly played with two counters increases the number of available options by much more than 50 percent. It is important to note, however, that the presence of the familiar rivalries, intrigues, and secret agendas of a three-person system is not sufficient evidence of movement into the Oedipal phase of development. A child may talk about or show in play phallic concerns that are derivatives of the drives in the context of basically dyadic patterns. In fact many adult schizophrenic and borderline patients create lives heavily laden with Oedipal fantasies in the context of dyadic relationships. Their wish to beat out father and to win mother is either in the context of receiving basic dependency support or in the context of a sadomasochistic dyadic struggle. These Oedipal-like behaviors are usually defenses against earlier, more primitive symbiotic issues of surviving and maintaining a sense of being loved.

One way to know whether a child has moved on to three-person relationship patterns is to determine whether he has sufficiently resolved his two-person relationship systems. Look at basic ego functions, such as reality orientation, impulse regulation, affect organization, mood stabilization, the capacity to stay organized under stress, and the capacity for an age-appropriate range of affects, including the ability to deal with loss, separation, and disappointment. A very subtle sign of having progressed to the triangular stage of development is the capacity to integrate life's polarities: ego splitting is not used by the child who in one lay session shows assertiveness, aggressive and passive modes, and hostile and pleasurable attitudes all as parts of the self. And the, of course, you look for evidence of genuine triangular relationships. Aspects of genuine triangular relationships involve affects of love, curiosity, lust, jealousy, and an emerging capacity for real empathy, as well as an ability to represent complex triangular patterns where the implication of any one move or behavior is seen in relation to both other members of the triangle. There are three variables in the system. The question is not "Am I loved or not," or "Am I loved enough," but "Am I loved more than him or her and will he or she be mad at me if I am?"

Next you want to know to what degree the child has mastered the tasks of this (Oedipal) developmental stage and resolved his triangular relationships. You look to see if his world of intrigues, rivalries, and competitions became displaced into other spheres—at school, for example—or if, on the contrary, there was some resolution that freed him for the variety of endeavors typical of the latency period. The ideal resolution is the gradual establishment of the superego, a psychological system that permits regulation of impulses as well as maintenance of self-esteem. You want to know to what degree the child's superego is internalized and consolidated; that is, to what degree he can regulate himself and reward himself for things well done, to what degree he has developed a sense of moral judgment as well as a sense of empathy.

If there is Oedipal resolution, and a capacity for self-esteem, then you are seeing movement into latency-age activities, such as the ability to expand from family to peer relationships, to focus on school work, to follow the rules, and so on. Peer relationships will involve the capacity to deal with a larger group. Themes of acceptance, rejection, competition, humiliation, pride, and mastery all come up now in the peer group. Find out how the child is functioning in each category described in Chapter 2, with a special emphasis on how she is negotiating peer relationships. Is she gradually moving from an all-or-nothing approach to her emotional life ("Everyone hates me because I got turned down for a sleepover") to an ability to see shades of grey ("Maybe she couldn't sleep over because she got involved somewhere else first. I'll call someone else.")? The depth and stability of peer relationships, the capacity to delay and cope with frustration, the emerging sense of ideals, and the ability to learn without sacrificing a rich emotional life are all signs of the degree of progression into latency.

I have been describing some nodal points, or milestones, of early development. You need to have your own outline, or map, of development, which should contain all the major lines of development and all the nodal points that you think are important. Use this internal map to raise questions about what happened in major areas of development. Obviously, children's reactions to the birth of siblings, toilet training, weaning, and other routine experiences should all be explored in the general framework of these developmental stages and model points. In addition, special experiences involving illness, loss, trauma, or stress should be fully explored.

In this section, I have not repeated the sensory, motor, cognitive, and language milestones outlined in Chapter 3. They should be covered in relation to the child's ability to master psychological challenges. For example, a motor delay and/or low motor tone may contribute to a child's feeling unsure about his body and therefore unsure about his ability to use his motor system to deal with aggressive feelings. A receptive language delay may undermine a child's forming the verbal aspects of his representational system or may, if he can't use verbal symbols in a two-way dialogue (i.e., no feedback), compromise representational differentiation.

What you want to have at the end of your history-taking is information on all the categories that we used for the initial diagnostic interview—the categories of physical and neurological integrity, mood, affects, relationships, communication patterns, thematic organization, etc. If you can develop a picture of how these categories of functioning evolved over time and at what point a child stopped operating in a developmentally appropriate way in any of these categories, it will help you greatly in your diagnosis. A child who stopped developing in a number of major categories (e.g., relationships, affects, mood, thematic style) at age 3½ is quite different from a child who progressed to age 7 and then lost some of his capacities to grow. A child whose progress stopped only in terms of the range of certain affects is very different from a child who stopped progressing in a number of basic categories, e.g., relationships, thematic organization, and aspects of physical-neurological functioning.

I hope this discussion has made clear how the historical perspective complements your direct observations of the child's developmental level in each area of functioning. For a more detailed discussion and framework of early development which covers both emotional and cognitive growth, you may want to consult Greenspan

(1979, 1981, 1989). A brief outline of the major points covered in the developmental history is presented below.

SUMMARY OUTLINE OF AREAS TO BE COVERED IN DEVELOPMENTAL HISTORY

I. Overall patterns in relation to developmental experiences
   A. Early homeostatic regulatory patterns (e.g., apathetic, withdrawn, hyperirritable, or engaged and interested in the world), establishment of rhythms and cycles, specific patterns of sensory hyper- and hyporeactivity, and motor tone and planning
   B. Early experiences of comfort, care, and protection
   C. Early feeding and weaning (from breast or bottle)
   D. Early attachment or lack of fit, style, intensity
   E. Early differentiating experiences and capacity for intentional communication
   F. Early experiences for organized, assertive, original behavioral patterns (e.g., in second year could the patient (P) engage in complex games and behavioral interactions? Could P take caretaker by the hand and show him or her what P wanted, rather than simply crying? Were emotions complex and rich, incorporating positive and negative feelings or did one polarity dominate?)
   G. By the second year of life and beginning of third year of life, representational capacities, as evidenced by indications of fantasy life, in addition to cognitive capacities for language, personal pronouns, etc.
   H. During third and fourth year, did representational differentiation emerge with reality orientation and greater capacity for self-care? Did this capacity begin to organize earlier magical thinking and/or regressive tendencies, such as extreme negativism or lack of impulse control?
   I. During fourth through sixth years, did relationship patterns expand into triangular patterns; did curiosity and interest expand (e.g., in the human body, sexual differences in the parents, relationships); did emotions become richer and more complex, showing greater capacity for empathy?
   J. Did participant enter latency, psychologically speaking, from the perspective of interests and wishes, capacities for self-control and regulation, moral development, school and learning performance, and peer relationships?

    K. Similarly, assess stages of latency to present stage of development.

    L. In addition, when not already presented, obtain data on the following experiences:
1. Birth of siblings
2. Toilet training
3. Initial experiences of separation (e.g., going to school, being placed for temporary/foster care)
4. Significant separations or losses (death, illness, divorce)
5. Specific family experiences or challenges (illness, moving, job changes, etc.)

II. Special additional focus (where not already covered) should be directed to the following areas:

    A. History of establishing relationships in the early years of life: whether P was withdrawn and very passive versus friendly and lovable; whether P formed intense attachments with parents or parent surrogates versus being "promiscuous" in terms of attachment

    B. Patterns of relationships with siblings, peers, parents as P was growing up, including exploration of patterns appropriate for each developmental phase (e.g., Did P get involved with other peers and go from parallel to interactive play? Did relationship patterns shift from dyadic to triangular and posttriangular patterns?

    C. Any major illnesses, including emotional illnesses, in P's life

    D. Development of affects and impulse control
1. Any indications of aggressive or sadistic behavior, or poor impulse control
2. Any indications of ability to experience sadness and mourning in the first 4 to 5 years of life or later
3. Comfort with assertiveness, passivity, and feelings of loss

    E. Feelings about own body, bodily processes; feelings and thoughts about sex; sexual experiences, etc.

    F. Feelings about sadness, hopelessness, "giving up," escaping, and self-injury and suicide

    G. Experience of child or family with drugs or chemicals that alter mood, behavior, or cognition

    H. Experience of child or family with physical or sexual abuse or neglect (If there is any indication of such patterns, pay special attention to signs of abuse or neglect in the clinical interview with the child—e.g., repetitive concerns with abusive patterns, promiscuous behavior, intense fears.)

TALKING TO PARENTS ABOUT YOUR RECOMMENDATION

Let us assume that you have assessed the multiple lines of the child's development in terms of age-appropriate accomplishments, that you have made a diagnosis, and that you have reached a conclusion about the type of treatment needed. It is now time to make your recommendations to the parents. You should know that many (some suggest at least 50 percent) parents do not follow the recommendations, often because of the family dynamics. It is therefore extremely important that you work with these dynamics as part of the evaluation process.

At this point, you already have an impression of the parents, either from your sessions together or from another clinician who has worked with them. It is beneficial to reassess the parents. Let them start off the session. See what their concerns are, where their associations lead, what kind of questions they have. Do not start it off yourself by telling them what you have found. A lot has happened between the first time you saw them and now. Let them bring you up to date: Have they seen any changes in the child? Have their concerns remained the same, or changed? Get them to talk so you can see where they are now. If they seem to have trouble starting the discussion, say something general, such as, "I expect you have some questions," or "Are there things you have been thinking about?"

It is particularly important to determine whether there is any parental resistance to hearing what you have to say or to the idea of beginning treatment, if that is your recommendation. If there is some resistance, focus on it. Do not skip over it. When you skip over it, you are just satisfying yourself: you are talking so that you can finish a process. If there is resistance, simply making recommendations is not going to break it down. The way to deal with parental resistance is to let the parents ask whatever questions they may have first. If they begin by prodding you, saying, for instance, "Look, doctor, we are just interested in what you found. We have talked enough in this process. Now it is your turn to talk," ask them to specify in more detail the particular areas that concern them, explaining that you want to make sure that you answer their questions. Tell them that you can and will describe the child, but in doing so you want to make sure you do not miss anything that is important to them. And again, as you hear them describing their concerns, you will pick up resistance, you will pick up denial, you will pick up distortions. Then you can talk to them about these issues.

For instance, they may have originally presented the child to you as depressed and sad, and now they say that he is happy and his only problem is that he is not reading well in school—thus denying their initial concerns about the child's emotionality. This is an opportunity to say, "I gather you've changed your mind. Your impression of him has changed from the first time we talked." And then they may say, "He is much better." You can respond, "Tell me about that. I am eager to know." If done properly, your comments will not be experienced as threatening. You are not saying, "Look, you are covering up. Your child is still sad and unhappy. How can you think he only has a reading problem?" You are not challenging the parents; you are simply a collaborator. You want to know how this child changed in their eyes. Maybe he really has changed. Maybe he was in a situational crisis and has come out of it; on the other hand, maybe the parents are employing denial and distortion. You have to help them integrate their earlier perceptions with their current one. If you do not help them, you are not going to have their support.

At this point you are constructing a bridge between the first session and the current session. Essentially what is needed is a restatement of what they see as the issues, which will provide an opportunity for you to work on resistance, distortion, denial, and so on. Encourage the parents to be as specific as possible about the child's original behavior, strengths and weaknesses, the child's feelings and their own. Basically, you want to help them with their observing ego because it is the parents who provide the observing ego for the child, particularly for the preadolescent. Whereas an adult patient brings his or her own observing ego to the therapeutic process, here the parents are the ones who will keep the treatment going if the child wants to quit. You want to get them to form an alliance with you on as factual and detailed a basis as possible.

After helping them overcome any resistance, your next goal is to enhance their understanding by giving them additional data. You can say, "Let me share some things that I have observed"—*observed*, not *concluded*—without even using the word "problem." You do not have to betray a confidence; you do not tell a particular content that the child disclosed. You talk about the child in all the categories that we outlined: the way he organizes communications; his physical and neurological behavior; the kinds of affects he shows. This approach helps the parents look at the child in a more differentiated way. They begin thinking of the child in terms of his emotions, moods, and activity level, as well as the things he talks about. You want to elaborate as rich and detailed a picture as possible, and to communicate in a way that they can understand and that corresponds with the picture they are trying to describe. You are helping the parents to be better observers of their child—a very useful therapeutic aid.

Again, you have an opportunity to see where there is resistance. As the parents focus more on the child's reading problems in school, giving mere lip service to the fact that he is also depressed at home and has trouble asserting himself with peers, you can say, "You know, we are both mentioning these issues, but I have a feeling you are more concerned about the school problems than about the problems he has with friends on the block. I am concerned about relationships with the friends on the block. I wonder why we have these differences in emphasis." This approach focuses their attention on their denial and allows you to see how much resistance there is. It may be mild. The next series of associations may begin with the father saying, "I was just like that when I was a kid. I also couldn't compete with the other kids and I would stay close to home." Often that kind of disclosure will serve to make the father feel comfortable talking to you. That is an example of mild resistance. In another family there may be immense denial; they may insist that the problem is the child's reading. It is crucial that you deal with the resistance for as long as it takes. If you cannot help them overcome it in one session, then see the parents two, three, ten times if necessary. Sometimes you have to see them repeatedly if you want treatment to begin; otherwise, you know they will not take your recommendation.

Now if you are in a clinic that limits the number of times you can see the parents, you may not be able to have as many sessions as needed to reach agreement on what the issues are. If the family is likely to flee because they are now denying that there is a problem, you can say at the end of the time, "Look, we haven't reached any agreement, but we have learned an awful lot about the child. I think we ought to take more time to share it. I can't be the one to do it with you, but I will introduce you to the person who will. She will have a little more time and can go over the diagnostic material with you. I think we should take as much time as necessary to understand what Johnny's situation is, so you can reach a decision about whether Johnny needs help." In this way you can delay the parents' reaching a decision while they bring Johnny in regularly for his "extended diagnostic" sessions. Even if they refuse to bring Johnny, at least the parents are coming, and you can focus on the diagnostic feedback for as long as it takes for them to recognize their child's problem at a descriptive level.

In other words, treatment, if indicated, begins with agreement on step one, and parents and child should not skip step one for the clinician's sake (so the clinician can feel his job is done and then say, "The family is resistant"). As indicated, therapeutic work can begin as an extended diagnostic consultation, no matter how long it takes. There is no such thing as an untreatable family if the family is willing to come in for extended diagnostic consultations. Helping parents describe their child in all the categories outlined earlier and comparing his behavior (in each category) in school, at home, in the neighborhood, and in the clinical setting will often be a very therapeutic experience.

When you reach some agreement with the parents at a descriptive level, you should then discuss the developmental level. Do not offer the parents dynamic formulations about problems of aggression, and so forth. These are not conducive to their collaborating with you to facilitate the child's development. Put the information into a developmental context, again using the categories that I suggested earlier. Show them where and why Johnny is at appropriate developmental levels or below in each category. Such an approach provides a nonthreatening way for parents to hear about their child's problems, and you can tell parents about fairly pathological things in that context. For example: "Your child relates to other people more like a 2-year-old. The way he clings to you and is very negativistic is more like a 2-year-old. There are certain kinds of experiences that may help him operate more like a 6-year-old." They hear references to age-level activities in school constantly, so such references provide an easy way for them to understand that their child has difficulties. Such a statement is certainly far less frightening than saying that their child is "disturbed": it communicates the same information, but more constructively.

Next, where possible, you may want to point out family patterns that are undermining the child's development and suggest alternative patterns that may facilitate his development, again using your clinical judgment about what is appropriate. Here you will most likely suggest areas for the parents to work on over a longer period of time in their collaboration in the child's treatment. Finally, at the successful conclusion of all this discussion, you can make your treatment recommendations. By this time such recommendations will be based on a common understanding and therefore may be readily accepted by the parents. After you make your treatment recommendation, listen to their associations for any further resistances, questions, or doubts. If you sense ambivalence, schedule another appointment.

Again, if you sense ambivalence but can no longer see the parents because the case has to be transferred, it is most important to recognize the ambivalence. Tell them that you sense they are still not fully in agreement with what you are saying, that you cannot meet with them again, but that another person will discuss the disagreement. Emphasize that it is best to resolve these issues before starting the therapy.

I cannot state too emphatically that step one in the treatment process is to gain collaboration at some level (even unconscious) on the problem issues and treatment goals. If parental distortion or denial makes such collaboration impossible, then working with the parents is the first and foremost goal. Parents who have grossly distorted views of their children are probably creating a maladaptive environment. An extended series of diagnostic consultations is the proper and excellent beginning in such a situation. Giving your feedback factually, with little regard for what the parents are able to hear and integrate, may take care of your need to complete the job, but in fact you are avoiding—just as the parents may be avoiding—the real task.

In summary, in this chapter we have discussed aspects of the interview with the parents. In addition to giving you an understanding of the "presenting problems" and past history, the clinical interview with the parents must be used to assess their functioning—both individually and as a family—and to deal with personal and family patterns that may undermine their "hearing" and following through on what we hope has become a collaborative set of recommendations.

References

American Psychiatric Association: Diagnostic and Statistical Manual of Mental Disorders, 3rd Edition, Revised. Washington, DC, American Psychiatric Association, 1987

Brazelton TB: Neonatal Behavioral Assessment. National Spastic Society Monographs, Clinics in Developmental Medicine 50. London, William Heinemann & Sons, 1973 (Distributed in the United States by JB Lippincott Co, Philadelphia)

DeGangi G, Greenspan SI: The development of sensory functioning in infants. Journal of Physical and Occupational Therapy in. Pediatrics 8:21–33, 1988a

DeGangi G, Greenspan SI: The measurement of sensory functioning in infants. Journal of Physical and Occupational Therapy in Pediatrics 8:1–21, 1988b

DeGangi G, Greenspan SI: Test of Sensory Functions in Infants. Los Angeles, CA, Western Psychology Services, 1989

Erikson EH: Childhood and Society. New York, Norton, 1950

Freud A: Normality and Pathology in Childhood: Assessments of Development, in The Writings of Anna Freud, Vol 6. New York, International Universities Press, 1965

Greenspan SI: A Consideration of Some Learning Variables in the Context of Psychoanalytic Theory: Toward a Psychoanalytic Learning Perspective (Psychological Issues Monograph 33). New York, International Universities Press, 1975

Greenspan SI: Intelligence and Adaptation: An Integration of Psychoanalytic and Piagetian Developmental Psychology (Psychological Issues Monograph 47/48). New York, International Universities Press, 1979

Greenspan SI: Psychopathology and Adaptation in Infancy and Early Childhood: Principles of Clinical Diagnosis and Preventive Intervention. New York, International Universities Press, 1981

Greenspan SI: The Development of the Ego: Implications for Personality

Theory, Psychopathology, and the Psychotherapeutic Process. Madison, CT, International Universities Press, 1989

Greenspan SI: Emotional and Developmental Disorders of Infancy and Early Childhood: Clinical Assessment and Treatment. Madison, CT, International Universities Press, 1991

Mahler MS, Pine F, Bergman A: The Psychological Birth of the Human Infant, Symbiosis and Individuation. New York, Basic Books, 1975

Nagera H: Early Childhood Disturbances, The Infantile Neurosis and the Adult Disturbances. New York, International Universities Press, 1966

Piaget J: The Psychology of the Child. New York, Basic Books, 1969

Index